HOUSE-TRAINING THE DIABETES MONSTER

R. GRANT FINES

UNDERSTANDING DIABETES

Learn to Avoid, Reverse or
Control this Horrific Disease

MG MEDIA

In loving memory of my father,
Royal Kenneth Fines
"I miss you Pops."

— R Grant Fines

CONTENTS

Forward. 7

Disclaimer. 10

PART I : WHY TAKE CONTROL OF THE MONSTER

1. Living Well versus Living with Health Problems. . 13

2. Metabolic Syndrome 21

3. Action and Intent 23

4. Basic Physiology: It's all about the Fat Cells . . . 27

5. Carbohydrate Sensitivity 31

6. How Much Sugar are you Eating 35

7. Susceptibility versus Pre-disposition 37

PART II : GETTING YOUR MIND RIGHT

8. Barriers and Filters 41

9. A Good Plan for Life — Be Active and Healthy . 47

10. Motivation and Habits. 53

11. Stress, Expectations and Taking Control. 57

PART III : THE EASY STEPS

12. Easy Steps Overview. 67

13. A New Mindset Towards Food 69

14. Weigh Yourself Every Morning. 79

15. Stop Drinking Calories 81

16.   Drastically Reduce Processed Foods and Sugar . 85

17.   Fasting. 89

18.   Supplements 91

PART IV : WHY IS ACTIVITY SO IMPORTANT? IT MAY BE DIFFERENT THAN YOU THINK

19.   The Benefits of Being Active 97

PART V : CARBOHYDRATE SENSITIVITY

20.   How Carbohydrate Sensitive are You? 105

21.   The Vicious-cycle 107

22.   Breaking the Vicious-cycle 111

PART VI : BASELINING YOUR WAY TO HEALTH

23.   Baseline Eating Habits. 117

PART VII : READY TO TAKE ON MORE OF A CHALLENGE?

24.   Restoring your Gut Health 123

25.   Determine a Normal Weight Range 131

26.   Cholesterol Ratios 137

27.   Alternative and Artificial Sweeteners 141

PART VIII : ALL ABOUT FOOD

28.   About Food. 147

29.   Meals and Shopping 159

30.   Emergency Foods and Snacks 167

Acknowledgements. 173

FOREWORD

I LEARNED TO DISLIKE diabetes as a child. I did not have it; my father did. Watching him struggle over the years left an everlasting emotional impression on me about this disease—an impression that continually seems to grow, influencing my entire life. I even decided to change careers and become a certified health coach in order to help people fight diabetes. And now I have written a book outlining the steps I successfully use in doing so.

The main takeaway is that each of us has a diabetes monster inside that needs to be trained or it will take control. The good news is that with some basic understanding and desire, this monster *can* be trained.

Nearly one in three people in North America have type II diabetes because they eat a diet too high in what I term "bad" and "ok" carbohydrates. Carbohydrates are well documented as the leading cause of type II diabetes in books such as *Why We Get Fat* by Gary Taubes, *Wheat Belly* by Dr. William Davis, and many others outlined in the acknowledgements section.

The following is from the American Cancer Society website: *Tobacco use is responsible for nearly 1 in 5 deaths in the United States. Because cigarette smoking and tobacco use are acquired behaviors—activities that people choose to do—smoking is the most preventable cause of death in our society.*

I would argue that at some point in the near future, eating bad carbohydrates will overtake tobacco as the most preventable cause of death, and if not death, then at least it will become the major contributor to a decreased quality of life as we age.

Each of us is different for many reasons when it comes to metabolizing carbohydrates. If you have, or are susceptible to, type II diabetes, then learning how carbohydrate-sensitive you are could be the healthiest knowledge you will gain. What you do with that knowledge will determine how healthy of a life you may lead.

Throughout *House-training the Diabetes Monster*, you will learn to differentiate between *good*, *ok*, and *bad* carbohydrates. In order to control or avoid diabetes, we must learn how much our bodies can tolerate. Continuously eating too many bad and ok carbohydrates causes insulin to stop functioning properly, eventually it loses its ability to regulate our blood sugar levels; this is called *insulin-resistance*, and it leads to type II diabetes.

There are dozens of excellent reasons to follow a healthier diet, but none of them matter unless we decide to act on those reasons. Once we choose to learn more, and possibly implement change, then books like this one can help guide us on a new journey and open the way to a new life—a life that is energized, healthy, and largely free of disease.

My approach to health coaching is to offer advice only when a person is ready. Advice and knowledge mean nothing if we're not ready to receive it. Nor do I subscribe to a one-size-fits-all approach. Everyone's physiological makeup is different. Our health goals are different. We come from different backgrounds and experiences, especially regarding activity and eating.

The first step I take is to understand a person's true health goals and what they are committed to doing in order to achieve those goals. There is no point in saying we want to be healthy while maintaining a diet that will likely result in type II diabetes. Take some time now to think through what your health goals are; even write them down if that works best for you.

I've lived a life surrounded by type II diabetes, which I will refer to simply as *diabetes* for most of this book. I am not a doctor, nor do I claim to be. My advice comes from my experiences and reading the books outlined in the acknowledgment section. My hope is you will find a few nuggets of information that speak to you and that this little book might be an opening to a long and healthy life free of the ravages of this terrible disease.

Good luck on your journey.

DISCLAIMER

The information in the book is not intended to be a substitute for the medical advice of a physician. Readers should consult with their doctors in all matters relating to health and for treatment of their medical problems. Although every effort has been made to ensure that all information is presented accurately in this book, the ultimate responsibility for proper medical treatment rests with the prescribing physician. Neither the publisher nor the authors take any responsibility for errors or for any possible consequences arising from the use of information contained here.

PART I

WHY TAKE CONTROL OF THE MONSTER?

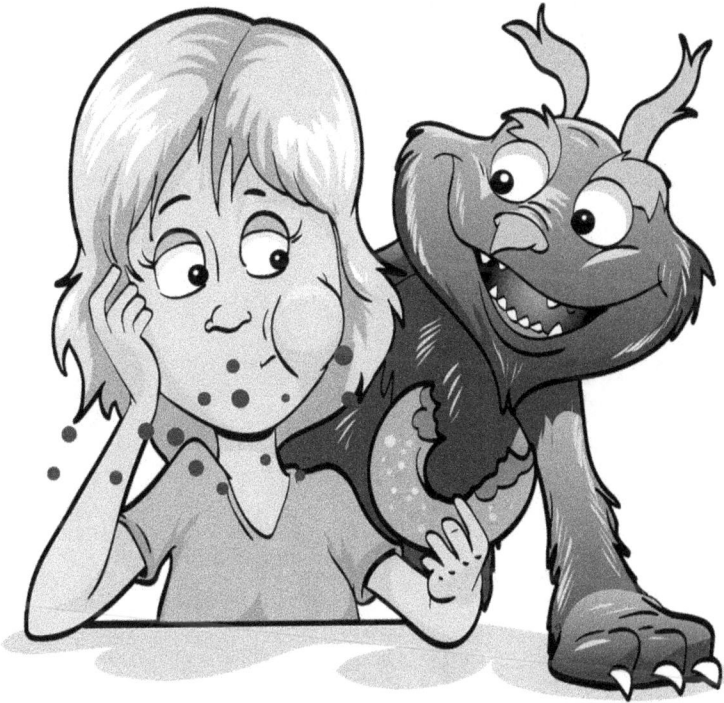

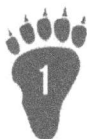

LIVING LIFE WELL VERSUS LIVING WITH HEALTH PROBLEMS

DO YOU WANT to live the healthiest life possible until your days on earth are over? Modern science is keeping us alive longer, and life expectancy has been increasing. However, what is often overlooked is the *quality of life* as we age. Many people develop some sort of disorder or ailment far too early in life, leading to a continuous downward spiral in health that can have a significant impact on the person and those closest to them. The good news is that many of our modern-day health issues are avoidable, and even serious conditions like type II diabetes can be reversed or simply better controlled.

What are your goals as you age? Is one of your goals to stay active in a sport, such as tennis or golf, or to be able to play with your grandchildren? Is one of your goals to avoid being a burden on your family or on your closest loved ones? That may seem a bit harsh, especially when accidents happen (when accidents happen, families should be there). What I mean is being a burden based on dietary choices. I'm not just talking about what you eat when you are in front of others; I'm referring to all of the things you eat when others are not watching.

Think back to five years ago. Are you the same weight today as then? Is your health the same? Are your markers for diabetes and metabolic syndrome, which you will learn about later in this chapter, exactly the same? If you can honestly say yes to these questions, then the next five years should be good ones for you. If you stumbled on one of those, think ahead five years. If you don't make a change today, what is your situation going to look like five years from now? How about ten years?

If you are ready to take control, then this book will guide you through the steps you need to make in order to live the healthiest life possible.

. . . .

Data from the US Centers for Disease Control and Prevention (CDC) in 2014 showed that more than one in three Americans are pre-diabetic, yet nine out of ten of them don't know they have it. That is 86 million Americans who are close to developing full-blown type II diabetes.

. . . .

The following chart shows the guidelines I use for differentiating between levels of diabetes. These are likely different than what your doctor would say, but most leading researchers agree than once your fasting glucose gets above 85-90 mg/dL, and fasting insulin gets above 5, you are pre-diabetic and without the type of intervention recommended through *House-training,* you will progress to full-on diabetes.

[1] GLUCOSE-INSULIN CHART

	Fasting Glucose (mg/dL)	Fasting Insulin (mIU/ml)	A1C (%)
Normal	75 - 90	2 - 3	5.7
Pre-diabetic	90 - 100	3 - 10	5.7 - 6.5
Type II Diabetes	100 +	10 +	6.5

I've had success as a certified health coach in helping people learn about diabetes. This ranges from those who are insulin-dependent, those controlling their blood sugar with a pill, those who have recently been told by their doctor that they are in danger of getting diabetes (i.e. pre-diabetic), to those who have a family history of diabetes and want very much to avoid it.

I remind my clients that it took many years for their body to become insulin-resistant and it will take some time to reverse the problem. Fortunately, our bodies are great at healing, including regaining our health from diabetes.

My first step is to assess and develop an individual's health goals based on the barriers in their lives. Once we do that we can formulate a practical and workable plan, most of which is detailed in what follows.

Determining your health goals is a giant step and one that shouldn't be taken lightly. There's no point in saying, "Well I want to be as healthy as possible!" and then do nothing until a serious illness sets in.

If you are ready, this book will help you form a plan to take control of the diabetes monster.

. . . .

Type II diabetes is a disease that centers on carbohydrates. It is a result of our bodies not being able to metabolize carbohydrates in the way it used to. If you can learn to properly manage carbohydrates, you will be well on your way to taming the monster.

Carbohydrates can be categorized into 3 groups: good, ok, and bad.

GOOD CARBOHYDRATES

These include leafy greens and other non-starchy vegetables, nuts, seeds, and berries such as blueberries, strawberries, and raspberries. These can and should be a staple in anyone's diet.

OK CARBOHYDRATES

These include starchy vegetables, all whole grains that are simply the entire grain, all legumes, quinoa, and all other fruits. If you are trying to control or heal your diabetes, then these types of carbohydrates should be consumed in moderation, ideally not more than once a week.

BAD CARBOHYDRATES

These include all processed grains, such as breads, bagels, cereals, and any other packaged shelf-stable food, plus all man-made sugars. These should only be eaten very infrequently and not at all if you are healing.

Go to our website, www.diabetesmonster.com for a more detailed list of all carbohydrates.

. . . .

When dealing with diabetes, I put a person's dietary needs into 3 categories: maintaining, healing, and control.

MAINTAINING

This is when you are at a normal weight, which you will learn to calculate later in this book, and when your markers for metabolic syndrome are all good.

HEALING

If you are pre-diabetic or taking a pill to control your diabetes and want to get back to having normal blood sugar and insulin levels, then I call this healing.

CONTROLLING

This is for insulin-dependent diabetics. It is possible that once you get control of diabetes and significantly reduce carbohydrate intake, over time you may be able to eliminate insulin-dependency. My goal with anyone who is insulin-dependent is to help them avoid health issues, such as poor circulation, kidney failure, and loss of sight.

. . . .

To most people, the word *diet* means something to help us lose weight quickly. That is actually the fourth definition according to www.dictionary.com.

The first definition of diet is this: Food and drink considered in terms of their qualities, composition, and their effect on health.

Here is the second definition of diet: A particular selection of food, especially as designed or prescribed to improve a person's physical condition or to prevent or treat a disease.

These two definitions are profoundly insightful because they address the impact of a diet's effect on health to prevent or treat a disease. Those two definitions should be the top two because what we eat has a profound effect on our health.

. . . .

I appreciate the saying, "When the student is ready, the teacher is there." Are you ready to be the student? There are a number of books and plans on how to eat and be healthier, but if you aren't ready to listen, or if they don't fit your beliefs, then reading them will be a waste of time. However, if you are ready to join me on this journey of learning how to be healthy and ready to fight the diabetes monster, this book can help you achieve almost immediate results in how you feel, along with preparing you for the healthiest life possible. Plus there is the added benefit of weight loss, if that is one of your goals.

. . . .

A defining moment that is etched vividly in my mind came in 1974. I was sixteen and went to see our family doctor to discuss diabetes. My father had been diagnosed with diabetes a few years earlier. His disease progressed quickly from controlling his blood sugars with a pill to insulin injections. I sat across from the doctor and asked him about diabetes. He told me that I didn't have to worry; that while it was hereditary, it actually skipped a generation. Young as I was, I couldn't believe that he was sitting there telling me that I didn't have to worry, although he'd just given any children I may have a health prognosis that included this new, horrible disease. The best thing he did was to give me a couple of handouts on diabetes. Although much of what was known back in 1974 wasn't terribly useful, the handout did say the best way to avoid diabetes was to stay active. This was reaffirmed a few years later when I attended the University of Victoria in its Physical Education department's inaugural year. Since then, activity has been a staple in my life.

I have been fortunate to live a healthy life by being active, implementing what I've learned after researching health and nutrition, and maybe more importantly, by learning to eat well, which can be monitored by one's blood work, digestion (which means how well we poop), mood, energy level, ability to think clearly, a feeling of being a bit off, and things we generally regard as benign annoyances, like skin rashes.

I have a passion for nutrition. Much of what I've learned has come to me via my mistakes and in finding out what works for me. You could call it a "sample of one." I learned that I had to listen to my body. I happen to have an intolerance for gluten (celiac's disease) and my body is almost certainly different from yours. But the basic principles that relate to glucose metabolism, insulin intolerance, and diabetes are almost universal. It is these universal principles that we'll be discussing in the pages that follow.

Our bodies are extremely complex, interrelated systems. Just when you read one scientific report that someone has figured something out, another report comes out to contradict it. What are we to do? Who and what are we to believe? Marketers are great at getting us to believe in something by changing the name, or using a catchy slogan to make it sound healthy and nutritious when in reality, the product is likely far from it.

Here we'll try to simplify the complex issues of how our bodies function with respect to diabetes and make those issues more understandable. My hope is to make it easier for you to make informed decisions regarding how to proceed, especially when it comes to eating and nutrition.

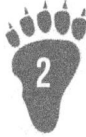

METABOLIC SYNDROME

According to the American Heart Association, 47 million Americans have metabolic syndrome; that is 1 in 6 people.

Take a moment and ask yourself how many of the following questions you say yes to:

1. Do you have high blood pressure, above 130/85 without medication? Or, are you taking blood pressure medication?

2. Is your fasting blood glucose above 100, or is your A1C test above 6.5, or is your fasting insulin above 10?

3. Are your triglycerides greater than 150?

4. Are you overweight with a tummy of >40 inches if you are a man or 35 inches if you are a woman?

5. Is your HDL level less than 40 if you are a man or 50 if you are a woman?

If you answered yes to any three of these questions, then you have what is called metabolic syndrome X, and this puts you at an extremely high risk for cancer, Alzheimer's, type II diabetes, dementia, non-alcoholic fatty liver disease, stroke, and coronary heart disease. Change nothing and the likelihood of developing one or more of these health problems is extremely high.

[2] METABOLIC SYNDROM MARKERS

	Ideal	caution	Poor	Yours
Blood pressure	120/80	130/85	140/90	
Fasting glucose	75-85	85-100	100+	
Fasting insulin	2-3	5-10	10+	
A1C	5.7	5.7-6.5	6.5+	
Triglycerides	<130	130-150	150+	
HDL	male >50 female >60	male 40-50 female 50-60	male <40 female <50	

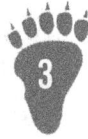

ACTION AND INTENT

SHOULDN'T WE ALL have a plan to live the healthiest life possible? If you answered yes, then what are you prepared to do about it? Are you able to take action?

One of my parents' favorite sayings during my teenage years was, "The road to hell is paved with good intentions." This was usually the advice I received after one of my failed attempts to complete a chore on time.

What stops us from taking action on our intent? It can be many factors from how sincere our intent is in the first place, to external forces that control our ability to take action. When it comes to making significant lifestyle changes, such as what you eat, or being active, it's those external forces that most likely are the biggest barrier.

Throughout this book, I will present you with ideas and suggestions on how to best navigate external forces and challenge you to define your intent.

. . . .

"We can put our faith in anything or anyone, and it can heal us. But the key to harnessing the power of the mind is to recognize that it's what we focus upon that matters—what we think and believe—and this comes from within." *How Your Mind Can Heal Your Body* by David Hamilton

. . . .

The first time my father's blood sugar went seriously low is one of those moments clearly etched in my mind, even though it happened nearly forty years ago. I can still see him stumbling towards his bedroom to lie down, announcing he didn't feel well. A few minutes later, my mom went to check on him and that is when my respect for diabetes took on a whole new perspective.

My mom yelled for me to come quick and I ran into the bedroom. My dad was lying down, awake, but completely incoherent. I could smell something like rotten apples. My mom ran off to call the ambulance and told me to stay with my father, not that there was much a young teen-ager could do. He moaned and shook his head from side to side, but no matter how hard I tried he couldn't snap out of it. I didn't think my dad was going to die right there in front of me, but I felt completely helpless.

The ambulance arrived quickly. They recognized the situation and did something to raise his blood sugar from its dangerously low level. In minutes, my dad became coherent, although he was completely exhausted.

The ambulance took him to the hospital where they stabilized and observed him. While we waited, the doctor told us what had gone on and what we could do to help him if there was a next time.

Unfortunately, there were a number of "next times," including when I came across a situation involving family members or others who had the same symptoms, including the "rotten apple smell."

I knew at that point when my father first came back from the edge, that I had a complete hatred for diabetes. But I also had the utmost respect for it. So far, nothing in my life has changed those feelings.

. . . .

As diabetics age, there are a variety of health issues they may have to deal with. These include blindness, kidney failure, and lost circulation to extremities. None of those sound very fun to me, especially now that we know how preventable type II diabetes is for those who are not yet insulin-dependent and how controllable it is for those who are.

If you are controlling your blood sugar levels with a pill, or have been told by your doctor you are pre-diabetic, then you can reverse the onset of insulin-dependence if you follow the steps in this book. I've helped people do just that, but it all starts with your intention and willingness to follow through.

For those who have been insulin-dependent for many years, your best bet at the healthiest life possible is to control your diabetes by eating in a way that allows you to take the least amount of insulin. Do your best to eliminate all bad carbohydrates and to limit ok carbohydrates to once a week. Just remember that any change in diet should be monitored closely by a physician and ideally with the aid of an experienced health coach.

Being able to travel as a diabetic is so much easier today than even a decade ago due to technological advances in storing and injecting insulin. That doesn't mean travel is worry-free. Insulin-dependence requires daily testing and injections; it's not as though you can just skip taking your insulin for a day or two.

Insulin dependence also comes with increased health risks including lost circulation, lost vision, and a higher risk for other metabolic syndrome diseases, such as stroke, Alzheimer's, and coronary heart disease.

It may seem an easier choice today to give in to cravings for sweets and treats, but if you think of the health risks of being diabetic, isn't a change prior to its onset a better option?

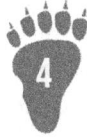

BASIC PHYSIOLOGY: IT'S ALL ABOUT OUR FAT CELLS

To BETTER UNDERSTAND diabetes, it may be helpful to understand our body's basic physiology. The following is a simplified overview.

What controls whether we become diabetic or overweight is mainly our fat cells, along with the hormones insulin, ghrelin, and leptin.

Our fat cells are either storing energy or releasing energy, that's it. By energy, I mean glucose. Our bodies want to maintain a perfect level of blood sugar. This is the amount of glucose circulating throughout our body at any given time. We can even measure the amount by using a glucometer. This balance is so important because we are always using glucose, even when we sleep. Glucose needs to come from somewhere if we are not eating, and it comes from our fat cells.

Carbohydrates metabolize quickly in our digestive tract into glucose. It enters our blood stream raising our blood sugar levels. In order to keep our blood sugar levels from going too high, which could lead to hyperglycemia, insulin is released from our pancreas. It tells an enzyme in our fat cells to pull glucose from our blood stream and store it inside our fat cells as a fat for later use, that's right, a fat. Our blood sugar levels start to increase significantly about twenty minutes after eating a carbohydrate, then after peaking in about an hour, they slowly lower over time, that is if you don't eat anything else.

When our blood sugar level returns to normal, insulin also goes back to its baseline level, and this triggers a different enzyme in the fat cells telling them to slowly release the glucose that has been stored as fat. Glucose is a small enough molecule that it can enter and exit the porous exterior of a fat cell. When the fat cell is in storage mode, the glucose combines with a fatty acid to form a triglyceride which is a bigger molecule and can't escape out of the fat cell. This is why when you eat carbohydrates, you store the energy as fat.

The other hormones of note are ghrelin, which you can think of as our hunger hormone (it sends a signal that we need to eat), and leptin, which is our satiety hormone (it tells us when we have had enough to eat). Unfortunately both of these hormones are dominated by insulin, and when we become insulin-resistant, it means insulin no longer works the way it should—that is when our bodies tip over to the disease we call type II diabetes.

The top graph below is what a normal insulin response looks like when someone eats carbohydrates. Basically, the level of insulin matches that of the amount of glucose in your blood stream all the way from when the carbohydrate is eaten through to when blood sugar levels return to normal.

The bottom graph depicts someone who is becoming insulin-resistant. The amount of blood sugar drops faster than insulin. Insulin knows it has been tricked too many times before by someone who continually spikes their insulin. It becomes resistant to getting back to a baseline level as quickly as glucose. Here is the problem: our blood sugars are approaching normal, and insulin is still elevated meaning glucose is still being pulled from our blood stream and stored as fat. If this continued for long, we'd become hypoglycemic. Instead, ghrelin interferes by sending a signal for food, and because of the potential low sugar danger, the signal is more like a mayday in order to get our blood sugar levels increased quickly. This hormone response is why we crave carbohydrates. This cycle repeats itself over and over. Not only does insulin not fall at a fast enough rate but it eventually stops responding to higher amounts of glucose. Insulin becomes resistant to doing its job. The Diabetes Monster is gaining control.

SOMEONE WITH IDEAL INSULIN LEVELS

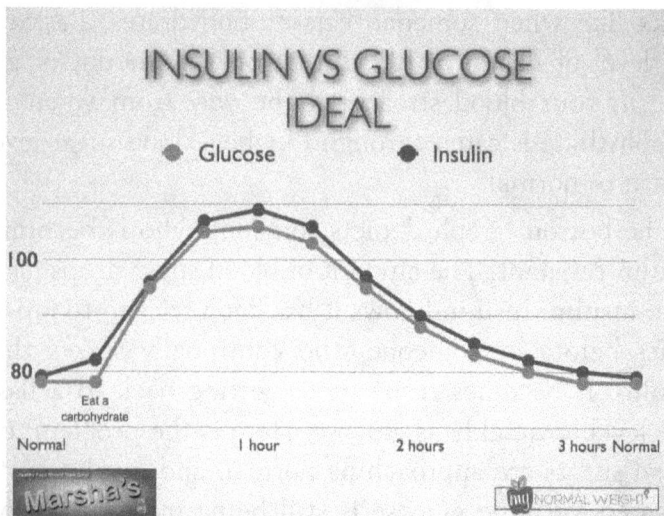

SOMEONE WHO IS INSULIN-RESISTANT

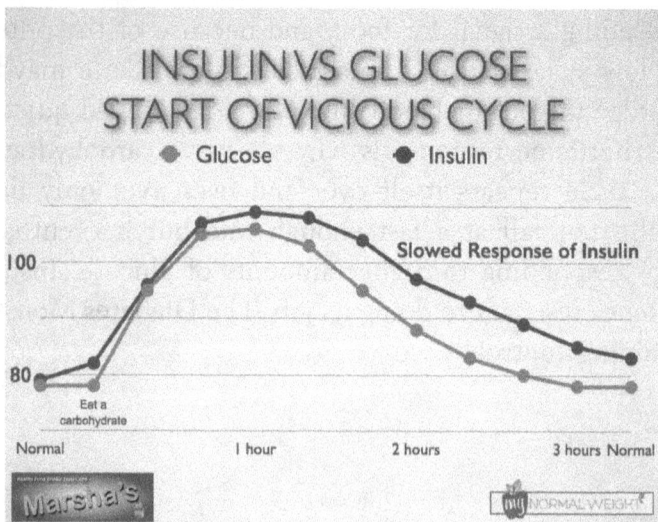

5

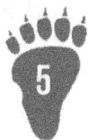

CARBOHYDRATE-SENSITIVITY

CARBOHYDRATE-SENSITIVITY IS LIKELY a term you have never heard of, but it could very well be the key to determining how healthy of a life you lead. Being carbohydrate-sensitive means you get a higher response from eating carbohydrates than others do. The saying, "A moment on the lips, forever on the hips." is truer for someone who is carbohydrate-sensitive.

Factors affecting carbohydrate-sensitivity include long-term antibiotic use, diets with bad and ok carbohydrates as a staple, being overweight, drinking too many carbohydrate calories each day, consistently eating past eighty percent satiety and age (since we become more carbohydrate-sensitive as we get older).

Ask yourself these:

- Do you get tired within two hours of eating a meal that contains carbohydrates (often referred to as "the mid-afternoon bonk")?

- Do you, or someone you prepare meals for, gain weight more quickly now than you used to?

- Do you still feel hungry even though you may have just eaten a meal?

- Do you crave carbohydrates?

- Do you wake in the night and feel like you need to eat something before you can get back to sleep?

- Do you wake up hungry?

- Do you prefer sweets and starches over other foods?

- Do you feel you need to have food with you at all times?

- Does eating carbohydrates temporarily lift your mood?

- Are you overweight, and have been for a number of years?

- Do you lead a sedentary lifestyle?

The more you answer yes to these questions, the higher the likelihood you either are or are becoming carbohydrate-sensitive. These may be warning signs that your body is losing its ability to self-regulate insulin, leptin and ghrelin. If you haven't had your blood work examined in the past year, including fasting glucose, fasting insulin, and A1C, I'd recommend that you have them tested now.

. . . .

Here is an example of how two people who eat the same diet, metabolize carbohydrates differently.

Marsha and I measured our blood sugar levels before eating our lunch, and both were in the low 80s. Our levels had returned to their baseline since we fasted for 4 hours after breakfast. We then ate the same meal: a salad with mixed greens, cucumbers, Marsha's amazing dressing, plus a nice size helping of leftover roasted turkey breast from our previous night's dinner followed by some dried apples.

After one hour, even though I ate twice as much as Marsha, including almost 2 apples worth of dried apples, my glucose level was 92, and hers was 105. What that tells me is she is more carbohydrate-sensitive than I am. Not that we ate a lot of carbohydrates. There were a few in the salad and cucumbers but those were mostly dietary fiber, and there were none in the salad dressing or turkey. The other carbohydrates were from the apple, which is mainly fructose that gets metabolized by your liver and turned into a fat, although some does get turned into glycogen (multiple glucose molecules strung together).

Marsha simply does not metabolize carbohydrates well. Not that a reading of 105 after eating is anything to worry about, but that is because she continues to eat a low-carbohydrate diet. It just shows she is more sensitive to carbohydrates, and she manages this sensitivity extremely well by eating a low-carbohydrate diet.

6

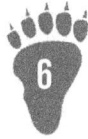

HOW MUCH SUGAR ARE YOU EATING?

SUGAR IS ONE of the most globally accepted foods. Its over-consumption is a leading reason why so many people are becoming diabetic at younger ages.

Take a moment to write down everything you've eaten for the last three days. Now count how much sugar you've eaten, including the sugar in fruits. You may need to refer to a products nutrition facts data to see how much sugar is actually in a product.

The average American eats between 100 and 150 grams of sugar a day. The American Heart Association recommends no more than 48 grams per day. If you are healing from metabolic syndrome and want to get control of the monster, target no more than 30 grams per day. That is the equivalent of having an apple, which has approximately 16 grams of sugar, a half cup of blueberries, which has 9 grams, and the naturally-occurring sugars in good carbohydrates.

How does the amount of sugar you've eaten compare?

. . . .

SUGAR = 1 PART FRUCTOSE + 1 PART GLUCOSE

Sugar is made of two equal molecules: glucose and fructose. These molecules are broken apart by an enzyme as soon as they enter your mouth. Glucose is metabolized into your blood stream, while fructose is diverted to your liver. I would encourage you to read Dr. Robert Lustig's book Fat Chance. His leading research walks you through how fructose is metabolized into byproducts, the worst being VLDL (very low density lipoprotein). This tiny cholesterol can penetrate and thicken your artery walls and according to Lustig is one of the leading causes of high blood pressure. If there is a bad cholesterol, this is it.

Products such as high-fructose corn syrup and agave nectar have fructose concentrations ranging from 55% to 92%. Your liver has to work overtime when dealing with these products. Surprisingly, agave nectar is marketed as diabetic-friendly because it is mainly fructose and not glucose, so it doesn't immediately raise blood sugars, or at least that was the common thinking. Researchers now know that fructose wreaks havoc with the control of insulin, which makes it very diabetic unfriendly. Please avoid using any agave nectar.

7

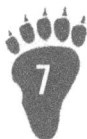

SUSCEPTIBILITY VERSUS
PRE-DISPOSITION

BEING SUSCEPTIBLE TO a disease is far different than being pre-disposed.

Most genetic diseases have a footprint that follows generations. These are diseases you may be pre-disposed to. Scientists are closing in on unlocking this progression, but for the most part, you don't have control over them.

Based on our physiological makeup, we may be more susceptible to metabolic syndrome diseases such as diabetes, coronary heart disease, stroke etc. but by controlling our diet, we can take control over the monster and lower markers for metabolic syndrome, reducing the likelihood you will get its associated health problems.

It baffles me why some people are so stubborn when it comes to what they will eat. Even with a health problem staring them in the face if they don't change. Part of this can be attributed to the addictive nature of sugar, artificial sweeteners, and processed foods which is why the monster can be so hard to reel in. Being able to take control requires "getting your mind right," and that is the subject matter in the next chapter. If you are unable to get your mind right about eating and lifestyle for your own reasons, chances are you will not be able to overcome needed changes to your diet.

RECOMMENDED READING

Why We Get Fat - Gary Taubes
Good Calories, Bad Calories - Gary Taubes

PART II

GETTING YOUR
MIND RIGHT

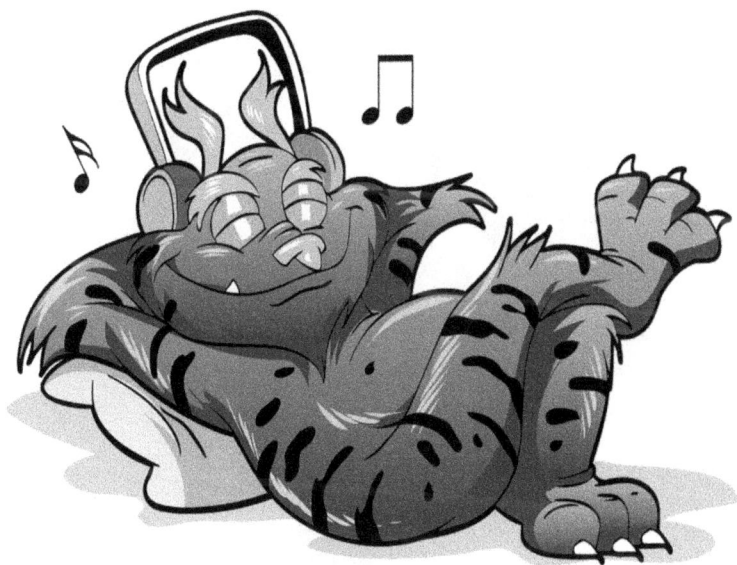

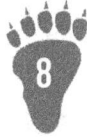

BARRIERS & FILTERS

GETTING YOUR MIND right could be a book in itself, and I believe it is the most important step you can take in anything you do. Having read hundreds of books during my 30-year business career, the ones I've found most useful were not the ones discussing how a business should function, but those that taught me about myself, how to take control of my own actions, how to navigate through decisions, and how to effectively get past barriers and to do things for my own reasons. That doesn't mean to simply barge through life with a "my way or the highway" attitude. It means we learn to make choices based on our needs and beliefs while understanding the needs and beliefs of those closest to us.

Getting your thoughts right is perhaps the most important section of any "getting healthy" plan, and this includes our approach to what we eat, relationships, our job, and so on. Those all begin with doing things for the right reasons, specifically your reasons.

BARRIERS

We all have barriers to navigate in our lives that include people, circumstances and thoughts. These have the potential to stop us from being who we really want to be, from doing things we want to do. Barriers can also be our generally good health since most of us take it for granted like water and food, that is, until it is almost gone. Only then are we prepared to do something about it.

Understanding our barriers is the first step to overcoming them. This can be challenging when one person in a relationship has a desire to make changes, possibly due to a medical condition, or to avoid a future medical condition like diabetes, but the other person does not buy into this change. How you deal with this situation can make a significant difference in leading a healthy as life as possible.

Remember it is not up to you whether the other person joins in on any changes. We may want them to stay healthy in order to maintain a great relationship and be able to do things together, but that decision must come from them. Sometimes the best we can hope for is that our decision to make a change has the others full support.

For the next few days, take note of all of your barriers and write them down. Include big barriers and all of the little ones, because they all add up. Separate them into ones you have control over and ones you don't.

Make a plan to deal with the ones you have control over and if you have too many, prioritize them and start with the easiest ones first. It may take time to get the perfect plan in place because of all the other directions we are pulled. You may need buy-in from someone close to you in order to avoid seriously affecting a relationship, but is this really harder than the quality-of-life consequences of diabetes?

For those barriers you don't have control over, it's important to put them into a good space in your mind. I highly recommend reading the book The Four Agreements by Don Miguel Ruiz. The agreements outlined in his book are great little reminders on how to keep life in perspective.

FILTERS

A healthy mind starts with healthy thoughts and setting filters to match your personality, your truth, and your beliefs. The thoughts we choose, or allow to stay in our mind past these filters, is typically what makes up our character and behavior.

That last paragraph could be very thought-provoking, or maybe it should be very thought-provoking as a first step to "getting your mind right." You may want to take a few moments to read the paragraph again, and think through what thoughts you allow to stick in your mind. Think back to yesterday: What thoughts lingered? Were you upset with someone or upset at yourself for not getting something done? Did you feel downtrodden because of how someone treated you? I don't mean an immediate fight-or-flight response to something that has gone bad, I do mean how long you dwell on it. Dwelling on it for any more than ten to fifteen minutes means it has made it past your filters.

Our filters tend to change through life's events. Sometimes we allow them to change a little, and sometimes more significantly. When we are the ones to decide on these changes, for our own reasons, it makes us who we are. When we make changes for someone else, it makes us into someone we may not want to be, and this does not always end happily.

We are constantly bombarded with influences to change our filters. These can be from a significant other, parent, co-worker, friend, an advertisement on television, something on the Internet, a preacher and so forth. It can range from how we eat or how we think, to how we exercise. Trouble arises when we change our filters to thinking or believing something we are not.

For example, if a mother is feeling tired and unappreciated, she may start saying to herself, "I'm a terrible mother." Even if no one else in the world believes this, if it is something she has repeating in her mind a few times a day, and if this goes on every day for months or years, this message will take hold of her mind and become her new reality. If left to run freely, this very often leads to depression. Even if the rest of the world believes this person is a great mother, it is what is in the mind of that person, and the tape that keeps playing over and over again, that can lead to serious illness.

I learned a simple trick to help people who play something over and over in their mind. Tell them to take the current tape out of their head and throw it away; replace it with a new blank tape that only accepts thoughts through a new filter. If the new tape gets jaded with repeated bad thoughts, it needs to get thrown out too. Keep changing tapes until one is found that only allows healthy thoughts.

Do you have a tape playing over and over in your mind?

Another trick is to say, "I can do this, because ..." You fill in the end of the sentence with what it is you need to work on to get past a poorly playing tape, or to help set a new reality, or for a change you are trying to make.

If a negative self-talk tape is allowed to play over and over, it "will" lead to depression or other mental illnesses. If you see someone spiraling down because of this, please seek professional intervention for both you and your partner.

It surprises me even in this day and age that going to seek professional mental help is still frowned upon. We will run to the doctor for the smallest of sniffles, but when the most important part of our body is misfiring—our brain—we don't get the help we need. There seems to be a stigma attached to going to see someone when we have issues with our thoughts. A good health coach can be incredibly valuable here. They do not replace a therapist or traditional doctor, but their goals are to help us navigate these types of problems by putting the therapist's or doctor's insights to work.

Another significant aspect to having a healthy mind is to eat well. Eating processed foods, sugar, foods with trans fats, and artificial sweeteners can sabotage a person's mood because of how these foods metabolize and affect our brain.

Getting our mind right, in order to change our diet is critical to getting past the addictive nature of these foods.

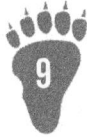

A GOOD PLAN FOR LIFE—
BE ACTIVE AND HEALTHY

RECENTLY TALKED TO a woman who told me she was diabetic. I corrected her by saying she currently has diabetes. By stating she is diabetic she's giving ownership to the disease instead of keeping ownership of her own health. We didn't talk much after that but I could see the wheels turning in her mind. I wondered if she was confused between being a victim and the work it takes to take control of her health.

Getting your mind right is the first step for any change to actually be easier. What I mean by getting your mind right is simply that we have decided for our own reasons to make a change. This is so important because if change doesn't come from within, for our reasons, chances are it is not going to stick.

We all have external influences that are both positive and negative. Some of those influences are with us daily while others are infrequent encounters. Only you have control over what you think, believe, desire and do with these influences. If the motivation to change doesn't come from you, and you alone, then chances are that any change that occurs will be short term.

. . . .

A personal story:

It was a beautiful summer afternoon. Random wispy clouds broke the endless blue sky. The air smelled fresh and clean from the newly-cut grass beneath our feet. We were sitting in the shade of my parents' apple tree next to their well-attended garden. Sunlight filtered through the leaves and we could hear bees buzzing and children's laughter.

The apple trees were laden with fruit for the fall harvest, and my parents' garden was in full production with fresh peas and other tender and yummy vegetables. My young children were playing outside, running, laughing, and enjoying spending time together with their cousins during this summer get-together. My uncle had come to town to check on his younger brother (my dad). A perfect family day, sharing stories and anticipating a barbecue feast that my mom was in the kitchen preparing.

As the afternoon went on, we were catching more whiffs of the goodness coming from the open window of the kitchen. It was one of those days of nice, warm, and deep inside memories that we hang onto.

I was sitting with my brother, my dad, and my uncle

on lawn chairs that were comfortably and strategically perched so we could keep half an eye on the children. Our conversation took us from childhood memories to recent sports endeavors of our favorite teams.

My dad's diabetes was partially caused to his physiological makeup but almost entirely due to his being overweight, along with a diet that included too many sodas. Now in his sixties, the effects of diabetes were really starting to take its toll. He still had his vision, but even with the heat of summer he had trouble keeping his feet and hands warm due to poor circulation. He was having a rough go at it this time, when we all descended on my childhood home for a visit.

Two years earlier, my dad had taken my then 5-year-old son to Macdonald's for lunch. It was just the two of them. He loved to do this with each of his precious grandchildren. During their lunch conversation, my son asked my dad if smoking was really bad for you. Not wanting to miss an opportunity to re-enforce the dangers of smoking to his grandchild, my dad did let my son know about the heavy risks of cancer and that people did die from smoking. At this point, my son started to cry and he told his grandfather he didn't want him to die and wanted him to quit smoking.

My dad never chain-smoked, but for as long as I could remember, he would have a few to several cigarettes a day. That is until that day at Macdonald's when he decided to quit smoking. A very powerful outside force, his grandson, had made him decide to stop.

Now we go forward to that warm summer's day in my parents' backyard. My dad had not had a cigarette since his lunch with my son at Macdonald's. I had just gone into the house to see if my mom and sister needed some help in preparing for the much-anticipated dinner and maybe to sneak a nibble or two of my favorites before they were set out for all to enjoy. When I went back outside a few minutes later and stood on the veranda, I couldn't believe what I was seeing. My dad had a cigarette in his fingers, enjoying every puff like he never had before. It shocked me to see him smoking again since I knew the reason why he had stopped in the first place. So much for that warm memory of the perfect day in the back yard!

When I asked my sister about it later, she said our uncle had goaded our father back into smoking. This made me wonder what it was that allowed my dad to overcome his previous feelings that made him stop when he was having lunch with my son that day. It took time to figure it out, but I truly believe the answer is this. My dad's decision to stop smoking when confronted by his grandchild was not his own. It was an external factor that led him to stop smoking. It was not his own decision. However, if he had decided to stop for his own reasons prior to having lunch with my son, then encounters like that would emphasize he had made a good decision. When he was sitting in the backyard with his older brother, he would have been motivated to say no because he had made the original decision. He may have needed to use self-talk like, "I can do this, because…' but his chances of saying no to his older sibling would have been better.

I use this example to show that any sustained change must come from within. It must be your plan, your idea, for your own reasons. Outside influences and information from others are good reasons to think about making changes, but you shouldn't make the change for the person that influenced you, you should make the change because it fits who you want to be.

. . . .

I wish I knew at the time my dad became diabetic to what I know today about carbohydrates. Keep on smoking and your chances of getting lung cancer continually increase; continue to eat bad and ok carbohydrates and your chances of getting type II diabetes will continue to increase. Keep eating bad and ok carbohydrates when you are diabetic and all bets are off for when some of its serious side effects set in.

I truly believe I could have made a huge difference in the quality of my dad's life, especially his last twenty years. This is part of the motivation to write this book. My father wouldn't be considered a good diabetic, but for a number of years he tried very hard to follow the advice of his doctor and nutritionists. Not surprising to me now, their advice didn't work, which is why he eventually gave up. With the success I have had in reversing diabetes, I know it would have worked with him too. The belief back then (and the mainstream belief now) is to count your carbohydrates and adjust the amount of insulin you take. This protocol baffles me because science clearly knows that carbohydrates, especially poor quality ones, are the root cause of insulin resistance. Why then would doctors say to go ahead and eat carbohydrates? I'm pretty sure they wouldn't tell someone with lung issues to keep on smoking and just adjust the amount of oxygen from your tank.

You've probably heard that when people stop smoking, their risk of lung cancer goes down and their lungs start to clear themselves. Our bodies have an amazing ability to heal. The same is true with carbohydrates. Removing the offending carbohydrates from our diet has the same effect as quitting smoking does to lung cancer. Our body starts to heal itself. We can even monitor our progress by checking our markers for metabolic syndrome.

Don't take this book as the reason to make a change in your diet. Instead, use the reasoning in this book to decide for yourself whether or not to make changes. If you do decide to make a change, it will be your idea.

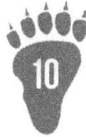

MOTIVATION & HABITS

MOTIVATION

WHAT MOTIVATES YOU? This is a simple but interesting question. What motivates you to get out of bed in the morning? What motivates you to go to work? What motivates you to do some of the things you do for yourself or for others? Do you spend time thinking about the things that motivate you? It really is beneficial to take time to reflect on what motivates us. This is what helps keep perspective in our lives. Take some time now and honestly answer some of those questions.

What motivates you to eat? Do you eat to keep your energy up? Do you eat because as humans we have to eat in order to survive? Do you eat for the sheer joy of eating? Do you eat when things in your life go badly? You may answer yes to some or all of these questions. The habits we develop based on our answers are important.

Many people are motivated to eat when there is a "trigger" event, this can be when something bad happens, such as after a fight with a significant other, or it can be when something joyous happens. Typically, eating after a trigger event involves pizza or a sugar treat like ice cream. Unfortunately treats sneak into our lives as a daily occurrence when they should really be something we have every once in a while.

If you are trying to heal from diabetes, instead of eating ice cream, try nuts and seeds, or protein like left-over dinner meat or perhaps a piece of cheese. Following this with a big glass of water will help keep your hunger under control. It may take a bit of time to avoid ice cream, but we can train ourselves with new habits and eventually this will be our new normal. A brisk walk around the block can also be helpful to avoid bad food choices, especially at night, and it's a great way to think through whatever it is that is bothering us.

Having a plan in place with respect to "quick foods" is important in order to make better choices when life's ups and downs get in the way. Having healthy options, such as a handful of nuts and seeds with a large glass of water, means having these nuts and seeds always available. Eventually, it will become a habit to check your supply prior to shopping.

It may seem a bit odd when thinking of our motivation to eat as being centered on something negative happening. We tend to think of being motivated as a positive, for instance when someone motivates us to be a better person. But motivation is simply the reason we have for doing something, or acting in a certain way. Understanding the motivation behind why we eat can be very revealing and also the start to being able to make sustainable changes.

Motivation is also personal. You cannot give or force yours onto someone else. Your monster looks nothing like your neighbors and yet they are both monsters. The training methods to control the monster are the same and can be shared, but motivation is personal.

HABITS

As humans, we are bound by habits. Breaking habits can be very challenging but also very rewarding, especially when a new habit like being mindful of what we eat makes us; feel better about ourselves, give us new energy, a sense of being the alfa over our *monster,* and can lead to a much healthier life.

The way we eat is typically centered on habits. When we need quick food, we have things in the fridge or freezer which can be prepared quickly, or we have phone numbers handy for take-out, or a fast food restaurant is likely convenient. The problem with these quick option foods is they often contain sugar in various forms, MSG in various forms, are almost always high in bad and ok carbohydrates and trans fats. This is why it's important to have good emergency food always at the ready.

Take a hard look at where you are at, and more importantly, where you want to see yourself in five, ten or twenty years. Are your habits today going to get you where you want to be? Are you willing to make changes?

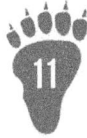

STRESS, EXPECTATIONS & TAKING CONTROL

STRESS

ONE OF THE definitions of stress I like best is the following: the suppressed desire to choke the xxx (you fill in the xxx) out of someone who deserves it. Unfortunately, we all have stresses from multiple sources in our lives that we need to live with. Having our mind in a good space is paramount for minimizing these stresses, or at least in minimizing the effects of stress, such as poor eating choices.

With the busy lives we lead, lack of exercise, and pressures from various sources, stress has a way of building, and it can result in an effort to justify whatever it is we want to eat. How then do we keep stress out of our lives? Well that may not be possible; however, there are things we can do to reduce stress. You will be the judge of what works best for you, but being active is universally accepted as a stress reducer. The effect of exercising stays with us long after the exercise for the day is complete. Other good stress reducers with respect to barriers are covered later in this chapter.

. . . .

It is vitally important to have good snack foods available when stress eating wants to take over. Keep these at the top of your grocery list.

. . . .

EXPECTATIONS

Another huge stressor involves expectations. This is a big subject, and I hope you take the time to see how expectations are affecting your life. Expectations come in many flavors—we may have expectations of our significant other, of our children, friends, family, church, work associates, what we get from working, what we get from serving in the community, and most importantly what we expect of ourselves.

When others put expectations on us, especially someone close to us, it sets up a potentially stressful situation. Think for a moment of what your expectations are of your significant other, a family member, or someone close to you. We all have expectations, and relationships seem to work best when it is about give and take. But how big are those expectations? How burdensome are they? This is about you, so be brutally honest with your answers. How much are those expectations you have of someone else setting the situation up for failure? How much are someone else's expectations of you setting the situation up for failure? Keep in mind these situations not only lead to stress if they go unchecked, they can lead to depression too.

. . . .

Spend time getting your expectations in balance; a happy future may depend on it.

. . . .

Managing expectations starts by realizing what your expectations are. That may sound easy, but it's something you will need to work on. Today, ask yourself what your expectations are in all types of situations. Ask what your expectations are of yourself, and what they are of the other person or situation. It's ok even to ask the other person about their expectations; this can lead to some very good communication, especially for someone you are in a close relationship with.

I would highly recommend seeking out professional advice if you are feeling stressed or depressed or if a significant other is feeling this way. I would add it is equally important for emotional healing to clean up your diet by reducing your intake of ok carbohydrates, and eliminating all bad carbohydrates and processed foods. Cleaning up your diet will be up to you as most health care professionals seem to skim over this part of the healing process. That goes for mental health and physical health.

We all have many outside influences with respect to habits we may be trying to change, particularly when it comes to eating and exercising. These influences could be in the form of a significant other, children, work, and so on. However, instead of these being excuses, these outside factors may need to be part of the solution. Working with these forces may not be easy, but we need to at least give them the opportunity to be part of the solution so they don't interfere with our "new" plan. Just keep in mind this is your plan for you, and set your expectations around this plan accordingly.

If you do get stuck trying to make a change, taking a trip, even a short one, is a good way to reset your habits at home. The reset works as long as you don't just fall back into the old norm the moment you arrive home. This again can require help from others whom you are sharing space with. They may not like or want a change, but in order for change to happen they need to at least understand why it is so important to you and to be part of the solution, even if this means solely as support. Remember, any sustaining change must be based on your own reason. Those close to you may not be ready to make the type of change you are ready to make. As in the example I used with my dad, if the change isn't your decision for your own reasons, it will likely at some point lead to failure.

TAKING CONTROL

Taking control of the barriers in our lives is not easy. How then do you get your mind right to help get past these barriers?

This will likely take a bit of work, but it does start with understanding the stressors in your day-to-day life, expectations others may have of you, expectations you may have of others which are not being met, and possibly the toughest question to ask is how you feel about yourself. Answer these questions as honestly as possible. Writing them down in a journal is a great way to get clarity on your thoughts, and will give you a record to review as you progress forward on your life's journey.

There are some things we can do each day to help. Taking time for self-reflection or meditation, taking time to put our feet up and relax, take time to observe and enjoy nature, and taking time to be active.

Self-reflection/meditation time should be a structured fifteen minutes, either at a consistent time of day or when it fits in. This depends on your personality, but take the time to do it.

To self-reflect, find as quiet a space as possible, no head phones and no music, and preferably away from any conversation. Do some deep breathing for a few minutes, four seconds in and four seconds out, this will relax your muscles. Slowly quiet your mind by thinking of, then focusing solely on, happy images. Allow the noise in your head to quieten down enough so you can hear only your own breath.

Once you can focus solely on your breath, imagine a serene image, then ask yourself questions which would be self-reflecting. These are questions about yourself, such as "How am I doing with xxx?" "Why do I feel like I do about xxx?" etc. Only you know the best questions to ask.

These will become more evident and clear the more you take time for self-reflection.

Taking time to put your feet up and relaxing is different than self-reflection/meditation and both are very important. Putting your feet up and reading, or watching TV is a good way to relax and slow your mind, as long as your choices are ones that allow you to fully relax and get your mind temporarily off of the day's events, or other issues you are dealing with in your life.

One of my favorite ways to "get in the moment" and to temporarily forget all the stress and "things" that are tugging at me, is to observe and enjoy nature. This can as simple as watching a beetle walk across a path, birds at a pond, or the different textures and colors within a flower or plant. Five minutes every day of getting lost in Mother Nature's marvels can really help put our life into perspective, or it can at least open our mind to thinking differently about problems. Why not give it a try?

Mental exercises like Sudoku and crossword puzzles are great at allowing us to temporarily forget our worries and cares. Forcing our brains to "think" is another key to living as long and as healthy a life as possible.

Being active daily can be as simple as a faster walk or climbing stairs, to structured time at the gym. As long as you raise your heart rate over 100 beats per minute for 20-30 minutes you will release endorphins and life will seem so much brighter. I'm not sure it is possible to get your mind right without being active four to five times per week.

The last point I will make in getting your mind right is about spirituality. I'm not talking about religion, or attending a church; I mean your inner thoughts on spirituality, on what divine sources you believe in. It is about getting comfortable with what happens once your time on earth is done.

Once you are on a path towards getting your mind right, for your reasons, then tackling some of the other steps in this book will be much easier.

RECOMMENDED READING

The Four Agreements - Don Miguel Ruiz

How Your Mind Can Heal Your Body - David Hamilton, Ph.D.

PART III

THE EASY STEPS

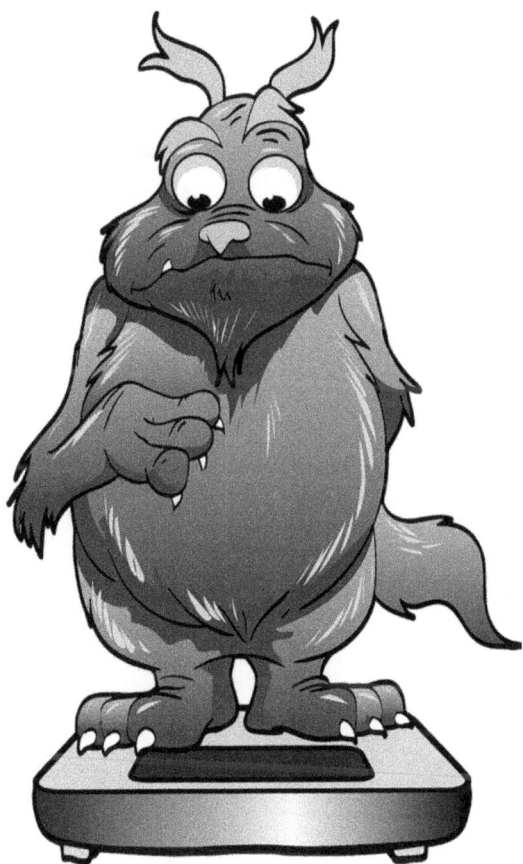

12

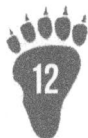

THE EASY STEPS OVERVIEW

THESE EASY STEPS become easier once we have our mind right about making a change. Take time to fully understanding the intent of the previous chapter and how it applies. Aligning intent with our beliefs and goals helps us to be successful on our journey.

No matter how healthy we are, these steps are designed to avoid, reverse or control diabetes. Depending on our goals and personality, we can start with one easy step at a time, or take them all on at once.

An important note is if you are healing, then having a certified health coach help you through the steps will make it a lot easier. Health coaches are trained to specifically do that. Plus making any drastic dietary change should be monitored by your doctor.

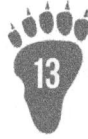

A NEW MINDSET TOWARDS FOOD

FOR MANY, THEIR biggest challenge will be to accept a new mindset towards food. We have been told for decades that fats are bad, but research proves that body-friendly fats as outlined below are essential for us to remain healthy. Making a distinction between good fats and bad fats is a necessity to avoiding the pitfalls of the really bad fats.

Recent generations are accustomed to eating for pleasure while ignoring the intent of eating which is to fuel our body. Eating for pleasure typically involves bad and ok carbohydrates, processed foods with all of their trappings, and sugar. All of these are quite addicting, especially to those who are carbohydrate-sensitive. When we start our day or our children's day, with sugar laden pleasure foods, we've completely lost the intent behind fueling our bodies, and it's time to rethink breakfast.

How often we eat pleasure foods should be based on our goals. If we are healing, we should have them far less frequently than when we are maintaining, and not at all when we are breaking the vicious cycle of sugar and carbohydrate addiction.

I find it interesting that once a person gets past their cravings for pleasure foods, they are surprised at how good healthy food tastes. It is very rewarding to me when someone says they didn't realize the flavors are so good in vegetables. This happens once they break away from ok and bad carbohydrates.

Another benefit to healthy powerhouse foods is we don't often overeat because our hormones are not being tricked as they are with nutrient poor foods.

Makers of processed foods know exactly what they are doing to keep you hooked on their foods. The potato chip makers' saying of "bet you can't eat just one" is catchy, but it's also true because of the product's physiological effect. It's really no different than cigarette makers who knew to put ingredients in their cigarettes to make them more addictive.

There is no one-size-fits-all approach when it comes to health and nutrition. Everyone's physiological makeup is slightly different, and everyone has had different eating habits from their developmental years, to the time they first live on their own making their own food choices, to today. The right foods give us sustaining, healthy fuel. The wrong foods lead to overeating, insulin spiking, depression, anxiety, obesity and many other serious health issues.

. . . .

HEALTHY FOODS

Healthy, sustaining foods are what I call body-friendly fats, healthy protein, and good carbohydrates.

Body-friendly fats

Body-friendly fats are mono- and saturated fats that include items such as coconut oil, olive oil, nuts, seeds, avocados, dairy, eggs, animal products, and wild-caught fish. Use caution when buying body-friendly fats because their source is important.

- Fish should be from cold water and wild-caught. I'd highly recommend never eating farmed fish, even at a restaurant.

- Dairy should be from an organic farm and animals raised without antibiotics or growth hormones.

- Animal products should be from sources that do not involve the use of hormones and antibiotics. Do you best to stay clear of animal products from a CAFO (concentrated animal feeding operation). This may be difficult because the majority of all animal products in supermarkets are from CAFOs.

It may be challenging to accept eating more body-friendly fats. We've been told for decades that fats are bad, and while there are bad fats, such as trans fats and vegetable oils, our bodies can't survive without body-friendly fats. These are referred to as essential fatty acids because they are essential to our basic survival.

A study reported in the American Society for Nutrition, was concluded in 2010 on 347,747 people. It showed saturated fats have no effect on cardiovascular disease.[1] That is a huge test both in the number of people tested and in the results.

Forty to fifty percent (40-50%) of a mother's breast milk is saturated fat. Why then, once breast feeding is stopped, do we stop feeding healthy saturated fats to our babies and children? The key is learning to distinguish between body-friendly fats and bad fats.

Healthy protein

The bullet points above on sources of fats are also what you use for healthy protein. Try to avoid products from a CAFO, and ensure they are free of antibiotics and/or growth hormones.

When possible (and affordable), try for organic animal products, including tofu, and if available, the best source of beef and dairy is from cows that are grass-fed for life.

Good carbohydrates

I outlined good carbohydrates in chapter 1. These are from non-starchy vegetables, berries, nuts and seeds, and are an important staple in everyone's diet. If you are healing, limit the amount of berries to approximately one half to one cup per day.

Balance

I outline my recommendation for a baseline diet in a few chapters, starting with a balance of healthy protein, body-friendly fats, and good carbohydrates. This means equal portions of all three, adjusting over time to fit your body, activity level and goals.

. . . .

Incorporating body-friendly fats while still eating ok and bad carbohydrates gives your body two sources of fat storage. Think of filling a gas tank with two hoses, one from carbohydrates (as carbohydrates store in your body as fat) and one from the fats you've already eaten. If your gas tank is the same size, it will fill up much faster.

. . . .

Inflammation is directly linked to health issues, such as diabetes, because it surrounds your fat cells and stops them from performing properly. This is another reason why insulin loses its ability to control blood sugar. It requires the fat cells to be free of inflammation to either store or release glucose, but when they are inflamed with a toxic blanket over them, they can no longer do their job. Eating bad or ok carbohydrates and processed foods feeds inflammation. Take a moment to let this paragraph sink in. Making poor food choices only feeds the monster and inflammation is one of the biggest hurdles to healing.

How do you decide what foods to eat and what to avoid? If you can picture the food item in the Garden of Eden, then it's probably good for you. Shop around the outside isles of the grocery store avoiding the processed and canned food aisles. Look for products that have one ingredient, or make sure you know what all the ingredients are. There are a few exceptions to those rules, but in general these are good reminders on how to shop and eat well.

Does it cost a little more to eat healthy, sustaining foods? Maybe, but that depends on how often you eat out, and on how much you value quality of life as you age. I've done many comparisons and we can cook a much healthier meal in less time and for less money than going to any fast-food joint or sit down restaurant, plus we have the benefit of feeling good from eating nourishing food rather than the craving swings you get from fast food.

Making more of your own meals is one of the best ways to keep the monster in balance. For some this requires learning to cook, while for others it is finding the time to shop and to get in the habit of setting aside ten to thirty minutes to prepare a meal. That shouldn't seem like a lot of time, however, when we think of cooking as a chore rather than an investment in our health, chances are we'll be eating out more often which is a recipe for feeding the monster. If this is you, then go back to chapter 2 and work on getting your mind right. There are fun occasions where a day is spent cooking, but most healthy meals can be prepared in under twenty minutes. Our website has a variety of quick and easy meals that do not feed the monster, and can be prepared quickly.

Keeping food alive and nourishing

Something to strive for is to learn to eat and prepare foods in ways that the food remains "alive and nourishing."

This may seem like an odd phrase, but what it means is the food is still in its basic form with all of its natural vitamins and minerals.

I will use an apple as an example. If you are at an orchard (preferably organic) and pick an apple from a tree, wash it and eat it, you are getting a food that is at its utmost at being alive and nourishing. Now if you purchase that same apple in a store, wash and eat it, the apple is still alive and nourishing although most apples have been sprayed with a wax to keep them shiny and fresh. By taking that same apple, coring and cutting it into small pieces, adding a bit of water and heating it until the pieces are slightly tender, we've started to change the basic makeup of the apple. When we make apple sauce, we typically use far more than one apple. When apples are heated, they become soft and will reduce into a sauce. You can change the consistency depending on how much you stir or mash them. Some items lose a lot more nutritionally when heated, but apples seem to stand up well.

Heating apples into a sauce concentrates the sugars and makes it a lot easier to eat the equivalent of far more than one apple. Added sugar or honey or other sweetener only makes it unhealthier.

When purchasing apple sauce in a store, be careful as it can contain added sugar, food enhancers, and preservatives. Even if the apple sauce is organic and only apples, the apples are concentrated and a small bowl of applesauce could be the equivalent of eating 3-5 apples, which is 45 to 60 grams of sugar.

Omega-6 vs omega-3

The ratio of omega-6s to omega-3s in today's North American diet ranges from 12:1 to 25:1 in favor of omega-6. This means we eat a lot more foods that have omega-6 fatty acids than omega-3s. This ratio has increased over the past 100 years when it used to be 1:1. The health risks associated with a high ratio of omega-6 essential fatty acids are inflammatory diseases, like cardiovascular disease, cancer, diabetes and other metabolic syndrome related diseases.

. . . .

Remember that inflammation doesn't allow your fat cells to perform properly. Do your best to avoid any foods that feed inflammation, such as products high in omega-6 fatty acids, bad and ok carbohydrates, artificial sweeteners, etc.

. . . .

Our bodies do not produce omega-3 and -6 essential fatty acids; we only get them through the food we eat. Both are important and are why they are called "essential." Omega-3 helps to build cell membranes in our brain, controls blood clotting, fights cancer, inflammatory bowel and other autoimmune diseases. Omega-6 helps reduce inflammation, fights heart disease, and lowers oxidized LDL cholesterol—that is if we do not eat too many. If we do, it has the opposite effect and promotes inflammation which really is the diabetes monster's favorite food.

The problem with the current North American diet is we get an abundance of omega-6 fatty acids from highly processed oils, such as peanut, soybean, safflower, sunflower, corn, canola and cottonseed. These oils show up in salad dressings, chips, crackers and in restaurant food. We can get all of our daily omega-6 needs from fruits, vegetables, grains and meat.

Excellent sources of omega-3s are flax seeds, sea vegetables, and wild-caught salmon. A high-quality fish oil is another great source if quality food items are not available or palatable.

REFERENCES

1 http://ajcn.nutrition.org/content/early/2010/01/13/ajcn 2009.27725.abstract

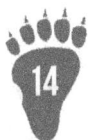

WEIGH YOURSELF EVERY MORNING

WEIGHING YOURSELF EVERY day is the perfect way to start changing your mind-set toward a new normal and it could be one of the best new habits to adopt. This daily ritual is the truth teller. The scale doesn't lie, although our weight may drift a pound or so from day to day depending on what we eat and how well we are digesting (pooping). The "time of the month" for women can also affect their weight due to water retention.

After consistently weighing for a month or more, you will start to understand what affects your weight. It differs for everyone. Look for trends over a few days. Are you trending towards or keeping at your goal or are you moving in the opposite direction? By keeping a daily eye on our weight, we can avoid seeing it jump 5-10 pounds before regaining control.

You will learn to calculate a normal weight range in Chapter 7.

. . . .

Poor eating choices can take a couple of days to show up on the scale. If you eat a big dessert and find your weight is good the next day, don't celebrate until weighing in the following day.

. . . .

When I eat at home and exercise regularly, my weight stays consistent, swinging by a pound or two. I am very careful of where we eat out because I have Celiac disease, but we have a couple of go-to restaurants. After eating at one of those go-to restaurants, my weight will be up 2 pounds the next morning and it is not because of overeating. There must be some additives or flavor enhancers they use at these restaurants that affects my body. It usually takes another day or two for my weight to return to normal.

There are other restaurants where my weight does not increase and I find this very telling of the quality of food that is used to prepare the meals. We don't always avoid the restaurants where our weight increases, but we tend to frequent the ones that don't first.

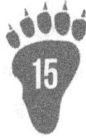

STOP DRINKING CALORIES

THE AVERAGE PERSON in North America consumes more than one hundred grams of sugar per day. There are approximately three grams of sugar in a sugar cube. This translates to the average person eating in excess of thirty-three sugar cubes per day. The American Health Association recommends eating no more than forty-eight grams of sugar or sixteen sugar cubes per day. I agree with that number if you are maintaining your health. However, if you are healing from diabetes, target thirty grams or less per day from good carbohydrates while avoiding all ok and bad ones.

A 12-ounce can of Coke and a 12-ounce glass of 100% organic orange juice have 39 grams of sugar each. That is the entire days' worth of sugar in one drink for those who are healing. By today's standards, twelve ounces is a small drink.

Our bodies cannot tell the difference between Coke and orange juice as they are metabolized the same way. Are you wondering about the vitamins and micronutrients that are in the orange juice or other juices? The sad truth is they almost all disappear with the fiber during the juicing process. Any claims of vitamins and minerals are from man-made ones that are put back into the juice as a replacement and these simply do not absorb into your body as well as the real ones do. If you really need those vitamins and minerals, then eat the piece of fruit and skip the juice.

If you really must drink orange juice, then squeeze one orange, make sure you get all of the pulp, and drink that.

. . . .

Starbucks recently introduced a new line of juices with no additives, no flavor enhancers, and no preservatives. The ingredients are simply from the earth, which is a good thing. One of the juices they offer is orange juice. The only ingredient listed is orange juice and it has been cold-pressed, which according to them is the best way to ensure the maximum amount of nutrition (minerals, etc.) is squeezed out of every orange. The label states this relatively small container is the equivalent of six oranges and the nutrition facts state there are three servings per container. Each serving has 26 grams of sugar. If we consume the entire bottle, which I'm guessing most people do rather than share with two friends, we put 78 grams of sugar into our body within minutes. This causes a severe rise in our blood sugar levels, and a corresponding insulin spike.

Giving up fruit and sugar drinks could be the single

healthiest thing we could ever do! It is far better to eat an orange and have a glass of water. If it's not possible to give up the ritual of having orange juice for breakfast, then be careful how much you are drinking. The equivalent of one orange is 1/2 cup of juice (4 ounces) which is 13 grams of sugar. A 12-ounce glass of juice is the same as eating three oranges.

A friend of a friend made a decision to give up drinking his calories which mainly came from Coke and orange juice. Instead he drank water. After a couple of months, he lost 54 pounds, getting back to his high school weight, and he is no longer pre-diabetic. He struggled for the first few days with headaches as he went through sugar withdrawal, but he willed his way past that and on to success. He is no longer feeding the monster.

Other non-caloric drinks besides water to consider are green tea and black coffee. Green tea is great for you because it has high amount of antioxidants. Matcha green tea has 37 times more antioxidants than brewed green tea because you ingest an entire leaf. A couple of cups a day can be beneficial. Watch out for green tea powders, especially in coffee shops, as most are nothing more than sugary drinks. Just because it says *Matcha* doesn't mean it's all good. Get in the habit of reading labels.

Coffee should be consumed black, or sweeten with stevia. Read the ingredients on the Stevia package to ensure the only ingredient is stevia. There are flavored stevias, too, which are just stevia and a flavor. These can be good to change up the flavor and smell of your coffee but make sure to read the ingredients. I mention reading ingredients a lot, that's because it is so important to not eat items that feed inflammation, especially as a dietary staple.

. . . .

Stevia is highly concentrated. When first trying it, start with less than the recommended serving amount as it does take some getting used to, but it is worth it if you like things sweet.

. . . .

If you have given up eating bad and ok carbohydrates, then putting cream in your coffee is ok. I recommend an organic heavy cream that has one ingredient, cream. Most heavy creams have carrageenan and this is known to cause inflammation in your intestines and is best avoided.

There are a long list of other drinks such as sports drinks and zero-calorie whatevers. My recommendation is to avoid all of these, especially when we are healing. These drinks are nothing but a bunch of chemicals that our body doesn't know what to do with.

The interaction of artificial sweeteners and the brain is far more understood now, especially their addictiveness and resulting cravings. Read their ingredients list. Besides water, you probably don't recognize any of the ingredients and neither does your body, and this leads to inflammation. These types of drinks are just as bad as pop and fruit juice, all of which should be completely avoided.

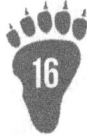

DRASTICALLY REDUCE PROCESSED FOODS AND SUGAR

OST, IF NOT all, processed foods are "dead" foods because the nutrients and fiber have been removed. The food has been treated in a way to make it shelf-stable for long periods of time and chemicals have been added to preserve it. Producers then add in flavor enhancers to make the food more palatable. The result is food which pleases us, but the physiological effect on our body leads to inflammation and resulting health issues.

There is a good reason processed food makers make their foods low in fat and high in bad and ok carbohydrates. This is what makes you hungry again soon after eating them, craving for the same type of food. Conversely, eating a meal high in body-friendly fats and low in bad and ok carbohydrates keeps us satisfied for a lot longer. Cigarette makers knew what they were doing by adding addictive components to cigarettes. I'm guessing the smart people who make processed foods know a trick or two about this, too.

. . . .

At the turn of the last century, the average person did not eat processed foods and they consumed on average six grams of sugar per day. Today, consuming well over 100 grams of sugar and eating packaged foods is the norm. These are a few of the many differences in our modern day diet.

. . . .

Sugar offers nothing nutritionally other than satisfying our palette. Because sugar has no fiber, there is no signal to our brain telling it we've eaten something. This is why we still feel hungry after eating it. The same holds true for the processed foods. Our brain has been tricked, and we want more sugar and/or processed carbohydrates even though we just ate.

I've already outlined how sugar causes our insulin to spike, and excessive spiking is what leads to insulin-resistance, and this leads to diabetes. If we need to heal from metabolic syndrome, then I strongly recommend drastically reducing your intake of sugar and processed foods and start incorporating more whole foods.

. . . .

This is a special note for grandparents, of which I am one. What a wonderful part of life being a grandparent, to spoil your grandchildren then give them back at the end of the day. Something I've observed with a number of grandparents is how freely they seem to give treats to their grandchildren. These treats almost always involve sugar and it baffles me why grandparents do this? You do not need to buy a child's love with sugar, you already have it. Review again the paragraphs on what sugar is doing to their little developing bodies and know that insulin spiking leads to type II diabetes and non-alcoholic fatty liver disease, which is prevalent in children today. Do you really want to do that to your grandchildren? I would hope you would love them enough to avoid giving them sugar. A piece of grandma's pie or cake has the same effect on their body as their mom's pie or cake.

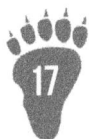

FASTING

GETTING OUR BODIES *back to good* requires a daily reset. To accomplish this requires fasting, and this includes a short fast between meals and a lengthy fast at night. The problem with processed foods and sugar is they leave us craving more of the same types of foods; we want to snack more, eat right up to the time we go to bed, and are hungry as soon as we wake up. By drastically reducing our intake of these bad foods, we allow our body to reset because we won't have as many false hunger feelings.

Fasting is the period of time between eating. It is how our bodies resets its blood sugar and insulin levels. We fast for short amounts of time during the day, and have a long fast at nighttime. Our nighttime fasting period is from our final bite at night until our first bite in the morning. If the last food item we eat is at 7 pm and our first bite in the morning is at 7am, then we've fasted for 12 hours. This would be an ideal fast! If our last bite of anything is at 10 pm just before we go to bed and then wake up and eat something at 7 am, this is a 9-hour fast, which is not so good.

The longer the fast, the more opportunity our hormones and blood sugars have to reset. If we are healing, then target nighttime fasting for 12 hours at least three to four times per week. Ideally, it would be best to fast for 12-14 hours every night. That may not be attainable right away, but is worth working towards.

Fasting for three to four hours after every meal helps our body to reset, especially if we are healing. This reset is something it may have lost along the way if we've been used to nibbling all day long. Eating processed foods or bad or ok carbohydrates will only make it harder to fast. If you do need a snack, eat some vegetables, or nuts and seeds, or a piece of cheese, then follow this snack with a large glass of water.

Fasting is a critical step in healing from diabetes. It is the only way our insulin and blood sugar levels can reset. It may be difficult for the first few days when we are breaking the vicious cycle by drastically reducing the amount of sugar and processed foods we eat. Persevere because it does get easier after a couple of days.

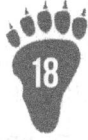

SUPPLEMENTS

RECOMMEND THE FOLLOWING supplements as part of the easy steps towards healing. These supplements are the same as recommended by most of the doctor/authors outlined in the Acknowledgements section. I suggest researching each of these supplements, the amounts you should take and possibly have your levels checked prior to starting. Taking supplements is a personal decision and if you are under a doctor's care, make sure to inform your doctor of your plan to take supplements.

Chromium Picolinate

This is best used if you are healing from diabetes as it helps to regulate blood sugar levels. There are two forms commonly available: glucose-tolerance factor (GTF) and chromium picolinate. The recommended dose for those healing from diabetes and metabolic syndrome is 1,000 mcg per day. Ideally take 200–300 mcg with three main meals. Take 50-200 mcg per day if you are maintaining.

Magnesium

Research is linking the effects of magnesium with insulin function. Magnesium is found in leafy greens and whole grains, but if we are healing from diabetes, then whole grains are in my ok category and should not be a dietary staple until our metabolic syndrome markers are all in their normal range. Supplement with 250-400 mg per day. Look for magnesium citrate, chelate, or glycinate, and avoid magnesium oxide which can be irritating to the digestive tract. My favorite is a powdered drink called *Natural Calm*.

Vitamin D

Vitamin D is actually a fat-soluble hormone and there seems to be no consensus to what your level should be. Based on my reading and research, I'd recommend aiming for a 25(OH)D level between 50 and 70. To achieve this level you need to supplement with 2,000-5,000 IUs of D3. It takes a lot of D3 to increase to this level. It is important to have your level checked, too much in your body (such as above 150 ng/ml) is considered potentially toxic and potentially harmful to your health and is just as bad as having too little.

Vitamin K2

Another fat soluble vitamin that helps our body control calcium and our blood to clot. Research suggests we need to take 200 - 500 mcg's at the same time as vitamin D.

Vitamin C

Vitamin C helps repair and regenerate tissues, protects against heart disease, decreases total and LDL cholesterol, and helps to neutralize the effects of nitrites. Your body will only absorb as much vitamin C as it needs, the rest passes through your urine; however if you take too much it can lead to a stomach ache. Typical daily supplement ranges are from 250-2,000 mg.

Note: Diabetics who are taking prescription medication for any condition should communicate with their doctor about any and all supplements and dietary changes. These may lead to improvements in glucose metabolism and medication dosage may need to be adjusted.

RECOMMENDED READING

Fat Chance - Dr. Robert Lustig
Grain Brain - Dr. David Perlmutter

PART IV

WHY IS ACTIVITY SO IMPORTANT? THE REASON MAY BE DIFFERENT THAN YOU THINK

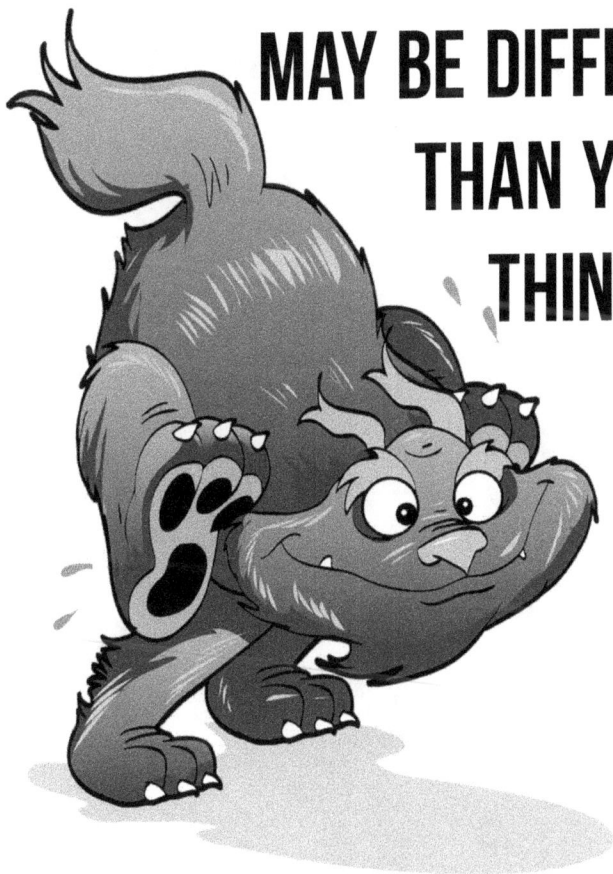

19

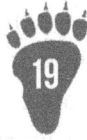

THE BENEFITS OF BEING ACTIVE

O NE OF THE keys to regaining control of our health is being active. Any activity where we sustain a raised heart rate for 20 to 30 minutes will help for a few reasons, that is, as long as we don't use it as an excuse to have a treat of some kind.

The #1 benefit to being active is it's a great mood enhancer. Having an elevated mood will make it easier to follow through on our goals and plans for a more healthful life, whether that is maintaining such a life, and especially if we are healing.

Another benefit to being active is that it puts our body into fat-burning mode, meaning the fat cells are releasing glucose into your blood stream to replenish or revitalize the muscles and other parts of our body that has just worked hard. Depending on the intensity of the workout, this state of extra fat-burning will last up to two hours or until we eat a carbohydrate. Eating any carbohydrates causes a rise in blood sugars and a corresponding rise in insulin which tells our fat cells to store blood sugars instead of releasing them. It's like a switch, by eating a carbohydrate right after working out, we lose the benefit of letting our body stay in fat-burning mode. Eating small amounts of healthy protein and body-friendly fats after a workout will provide the needed amino and fatty acids for repairing muscles and tissue from our workout. We simply don't need the carbohydrates.

I like using the word *activity* instead of *exercise*, although I do interchange them. When people think of exercise, they think gym memberships, the latest workout gear, and structured class workouts. Those work great, but so does a brisk walk, running around with children for an hour, or any form of activity that sustains our heart rate depending on our physical condition. If you have not been active for any length of time, then I highly recommend seeing a doctor prior to starting any new activity, then start slow and work your way up. Ideally we should be active 4-5 times a week for 20-30 minutes of sustained elevated heart rate based on your physical condition.

Notice so far I haven't mentioned weight loss as a result from being active. It can happen, but we have to exercise a lot every day for this to happen. Weight loss is best accomplished by regulating what we eat, and using activity to keep our mood elevated in order to not cheat when eating.

．．．．．．．．．．

I co-hosted a TV show entitled "Sport Fishing on the Fly" with Don Freschi. It was a how-to television series on fly fishing. On one particular trip, we were allowed access to film an episode at a farmer's pond which he had stocked a few years past. The fish were rainbow trout. They were huge and we had a blast catching and filming these "giant toads" as we referred to them on the show. While we fished I enjoyed watching the farmer work his land on his tractor. Near noon, he stopped his tractor near a dirt road. I was anticipating that he was going to get out and eat his lunch. Instead, he climbed out of the cab of his tractor, did a few stretches, and started off jogging down the dirt road. Almost an hour later, the farmer returned, still jogging back to his tractor. He stretched for a few minutes, climbed back into the cab and started working his field again. No gym, no special shoes, no ceremony. Just something he did for his reasons, but what a very inspiring sight to see.

. . . .

I had been training for my upcoming triathlon season a few years ago, and my body weight of 172 pounds seemed perfect for the rigors of a triathlon. During a training ride two weeks before my first one, an ignorant soul ran me off the road while I rode my tri-bike (not a tricycle). I was doing 25 miles per hour and the resulting crash left me with a severely bruised wrist and knee, over a dozen stitches, and plenty of road rash, but fortunately nothing broken. I had to take six weeks off of training. Can you guess what my weight was after six weeks of complete inactivity? I'll tell you in a paragraph.

A few years later, I decided to try and complete another marathon, as our schedule allowed me to do the tedious training. I had a great base to start and had increased my long training runs to over 12 miles. Then my knee flared up. I tried to run through it, but after a couple of weeks, I decided it wasn't worth a chronic injury just to complete another marathon. I shut down my running, and gave my body a complete break from all activity. Six weeks later, I resumed jogging and some mild activity to wake my body back up. I weighed 171 pounds when my knee acted up. Can you guess what my weight was after another six weeks of inactivity?

Before my bike accident, I weighed 172 pounds; six weeks later with no activity, I weighed 170 pounds, down two pounds from my training weight. Six weeks after my knee injury from running, my weight was 172 pounds, up one pound.

I hope this shows that while activity is an important part of a living healthy plan, what we eat is far more important than how much we exercise.

How was I able to maintain my weight during those six weeks of complete inactivity? I just stopped eating, right? Well, not exactly, although I did cut my caloric intake from 3,200 calories per day to 1,800. My activity level went from two hours per day to zero. My immediate mind-set upon being injured was to give my body what it needed to help in healing. The significant change I made was to cut out all ok and bad carbohydrates while increasing my intake of body-friendly fats and healthy protein. Having a diet higher in these helped to heal my body. Eating carbohydrates and sugar would have left me feeling hungry and I didn't need this feeling while sitting around the house, plus they promote and feed the inflammation which is what my body was now battling.

. . . .

An interesting myth is that with a little hard work and some weight training, you can turn fat into muscle. Fat, however, is not a protein and there is no mechanism for it to turn into one. You can only reduce the amount of fat by changing your diet, and you can only increase the amount of muscle by exercising.

. . . .

Marsha and I recently went to cheer on the finishers at an Ironman competition. I've watched a few friends train for and do well in these competitions, but it's not something I've felt compelled to accomplish in my lifetime. Marsha asked a question as we watched, "What could be so horribly wrong in someone's life that they would subject themselves to this type of hell for 12 plus hours and all the training to get ready for it?" This comment really made me think, and to question a few athletes. For some it was just an extension of the training they had done their entire lives. For others it was to change the way they approached life. Ten athletes gave 10 different answers.

Marsha's question made me wonder, "What could be so horribly wrong in someone's life that they allow themselves to eat poorly and continually spike their insulin when they know the implications for themselves and those around them as they age?"

I'm sure there are a million answers to that question, but I believe an honest answer is one of the keys to building a resistance to eating poorly and dealing with diabetes. I'd add that being honest needs to transcend to someone else if they are part of "what is wrong." Being active is one of the best ways to help build the resistance.

RECOMMENDED READING

PACE: Rediscover Your Native Fitness - Dr. Al Sears

PART V

CARBOHYDRATE SENSITIVITY

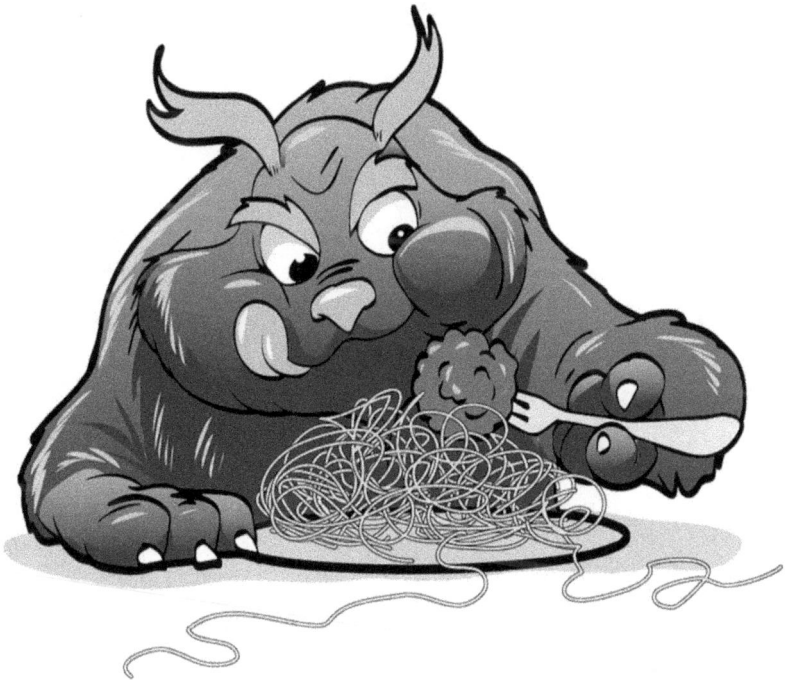

20

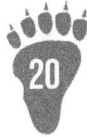

HOW CARBOHYDRATE-SENSITIVE ARE YOU?

CARBOHYDRATE SENSITIVITY IS not a medical term but one that is used to describe how sensitive some people's bodies are at metabolizing carbohydrates. Some of us are physiologically more prone to carbohydrate sensitivity, while others train their bodies to be like this from years of eating bad and ok carbohydrates. There is also a link between excessive antibiotic use and carbohydrate sensitivity.

Dr. Paul Navar used to warn his female patients that once they reach age 40, they need to cut down on the carbohydrates they have as a staple in their diet because of being more carbohydrate sensitive as they age.

Most of us have heard someone say, "I exercise the same and eat the same, yet I've put on weight." For a lot of us, this means an expanded tummy because of our body's inability to effectively deal with carbohydrates. The solution is to eat less ok and bad carbohydrates. Men also become more carbohydrate-sensitive as they age, partly due to being less active and a link between this and hormone levels.

You may want to review the list of questions in Chapter One on carbohydrate sensitivity.

Becoming carbohydrate-sensitive is also an indicator you may becoming insulin-resistant. If you haven't had your blood work done in over a year, now would be a good time. Compare your results to the chart at the beginning of this book and make sure your doctor orders a fasting insulin test.

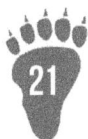

THE VICIOUS CYCLE

THE MORE CARBOHYDRATE-SENSITIVE we are, the quicker we may become insulin-resistant—that is, unless we give up eating bad and ok carbohydrates as a staple in our diet.

As our blood sugar levels return to normal after eating, insulin should also return to normal. If we are insulin-resistant, insulin remains above its baseline. Our fat cells still get the message to pull glucose from our blood stream and store it as fat. This causes our blood sugar levels to continually drop and is a recipe for hypoglycemia, or low blood sugar. This is when leptin and ghrelin send a signal telling our brain about the potential low blood sugar and something needs to happen, and it better be quick. Think of it more as a mayday or distress signal. The signal is actually a craving for carbohydrates which our body knows metabolizes quickly to blood sugar, in order to prevent hypoglycemic.

If we give in and eat carbohydrates, our blood sugars rise along with insulin. Our body will use a small percent of the new glucose but the rest will continue to be stored inside our fat cells because insulin is still telling them to do this. Over time, our blood sugars will return to normal, but insulin is resistant to going back to its normal level and the cycle repeats over and over.

Eventually insulin just gives up trying to regulate at all. This is when we become a pill- or insulin-dependent type II diabetic.

. . . .

Marsha is far more carbohydrate-sensitive than I am and maybe more significant is the major cravings she gets when she eats carbohydrates. These cravings are almost impossible for her to ignore because she is quite carbohydrate-sensitive. This is why she has decided to keep them completely out of her diet and has her *mind right* as outlined in Chapter 2.

We work together in our house to make it easy. We have a completely gluten free house even though Marsha is not Celiac, and we rarely have bad or ok carbohydrates because of how carbohydrate sensitive she is.

. . . .

For most people, once you become carbohydrate-sensitive, removing carbohydrates as a staple in your diet is the only way to avoid its pitfalls; weight gain, cravings for more and more carbohydrates that becomes a vicious cycle, and ultimately when your body finally exhausts its ability to regulate insulin, you become a type II diabetic.

Unfortunately in this day and age of diets that are high in sugar and processed foods, even young children are becoming carbohydrate-sensitive, and fatty liver disease is growing at an alarming rate. Please be mindful if you are feeding a child!

. . . .

Moore's law of technological doubling every 18-24 months is what Intel has used as its competitive advantage. This increase in technology has allowed the medical industry some great insight into the human body because they now have the tools to see smaller and peer deeper which enhances and, in some cases, enables research. These new tools will continue to evolve, as will our understanding of the human body and all of the physiological effects it undergoes.

Being proactive is so important. If we wait for the government to catch up and adjust their stance on our dietary needs, we won't take advantage of the new research which enables us to achieve the best lives that we can. Think how long it took the government to force cigarette makers to remove all advertising and include serious health warnings on the packaging. I can see a day coming when they will do the same to sugar and processed foods.

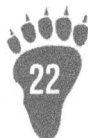

BREAKING THE VICIOUS CYCLE

REAKING THE VICIOUS cycle requires getting past cravings for sugar and processed foods. The best way I've found to accomplish this is by completely eliminating them, even as a snack and/or treat. Once the cycle is broken, then it's up to you to decide how much you put back into your diet. Just remember they are addictive and can cause recidivism unless you have the intestinal fortitude to be strong. Remember your saying, "I can do this, because…"

The physiological effects for the first few days of eliminating these foods include headaches, major cravings, irritability, and longing for your old habits. If you can persevere without giving in, these effects get easier.

Strategies

- Make a plan for 4-5 days of exactly what you are going to eat for meals and snacks (refer to chapter 8 for meal ideas). Go to the store and buy everything you need for these first days to avoid being in the store when you are hungry or having cravings.

- Ensure you have plenty of healthy snacks available (see the recommended snack list in chapter 8) because cravings could be your biggest undoing.

- Drink plenty of water each day. Drinking a glass after a healthy snack can help you feel full.

- Fast for 12 hours each night. This critical step may be the hardest part because it requires no nighttime eating.

- Fast a minimum of two hours after each meal. Do your best to stretch your after-meal fast to three hours.

- Start each morning with a large glass of water.

- Do your best to not eat the moment you wake up, instead try some meditation, or light stretching, or yoga, or go for a walk around the block. Have a morning drink of black coffee or unsweetened tea, and then eat your breakfast.

- Eat only foods from the list of good carbohydrates, healthy protein and body friendly fats.

- Be active, but do not exercise vigorously. Walks, especially at night when the pantry is calling, can help stave off a snacking setback. The longer we go without sugar and processed foods, the easier it gets, but giving in, even for one item can set us back 2 steps.

RECOMMENDED READING

Clean - Dr. Alejandro Junger
Beat Sugar Addiction Now - Dr. Jacob Teitelbaum

PART VI

BASELINING YOUR WAY TO HEALTH

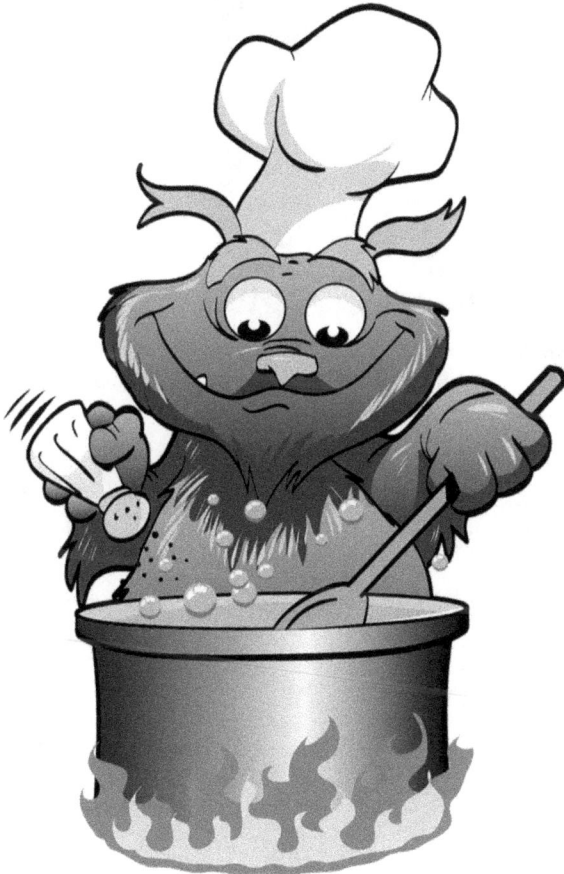

23

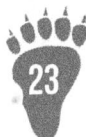

BASELINE EATING HABITS

BASELINE EATING REFERS to all of the foods we eat as a staple. Solid baseline eating habits gives us something to fall back on when eating gets out of control due to family functions, work, life, holidays, and so forth. Having great baseline eating habits is like having a perfect reset button, allowing us to get back to good after a few days of baseline eating.

Your baseline is what you eat as a staple every one to three days and should include healthy protein, body-friendly fats, and good carbohydrates. The ratio of these is dependent on your physiological makeup, your activity level, how carbohydrate-sensitive you are, if you are healing or maintaining, and what your desires and expectations are about food.

Our baseline is our go-to everyday food; it's what we have in our fridge, pantry, cupboards and freezer. The final chapter in this book outlines some good choices.

If you eat ice cream a few times a week, then this is part of your baseline and right now would be a good time to decide if it's in your best interest to continue with some of the foods you have as a staple, like ice cream.

The hardest decision will likely be deciding how much and how often to include ok carbohydrates. As I've stated throughout, if you are healing, then consider none to be your best way forward—use them as a weekly treat instead of a baseline. If you are maintaining, then determine how carbohydrate-sensitive you are, and keep in mind what the future consequences may be from eating ok carbohydrates.

. . . .

Shortly after lunch, I was visiting my very overweight lawyer regarding our business. He spoke openly to me about his weight issue knowing I was a certified health coach. He had joined one of those weight loss programs which sends you pre-packaged food in the mail (read again my dislike for processed foods). On this day he had forgotten to bring his pre-packaged lunch, so he went to the local grocery store and quite proudly announced that he had only eaten a baked potato with broccoli and he skipped the cheese.

My reaction was much less than he had hoped. I had to explain that the potato was like eating a bowl of sugar because it was all carbohydrates and would spike his insulin severely. While he did get a bit of fiber and some micro nutrients, his goal was weight loss and reversal from diabetes. The baked potato, which I put on my ok carbo-hydrate list, did not help achieve his goal because he was healing and should avoid all ok and bad carbs. His blood sugar would have spiked after his lunch, and depending on his insulin's level of resistance, it would have spiked too. Based on his pre-diabetic condition and the vicious cycle I outlined earlier, his insulin would likely lag well behind his blood sugar. After a blood sugar high, he would have had to deal with a severe blood sugar low and he would have had hunger pangs all afternoon, that is, until he gave in to eating something else.

Choosing broccoli was obviously good. Skipping the cheese sauce was probably also good because it was likely made with bad fats instead of body-friendly fats, plus it likely had sugar in it to mask the poor ingredients.

Instead of the baked potato, he should have eaten a piece of protein, like a chicken breast, some vegetables, and some leafy greens (using olive oil as the base for his salad dressing). The piece of protein could even have been a good-sized portion to help sustain him until his nighttime meal. He wouldn't have had any insulin spiking from this type of meal, and he would have made it a lot longer before feeling hungry. Then when his hunger did come on, he could eat a handful of walnuts or pecans and a glass of water to get him through until dinner. This type of meal and snack would not raise his blood sugar level, nor would it spike his insulin level. Plus he would feel satisfied after eating and could fast for a longer interval than his baked potato choice.

. . . .

I use this example because it's a scenario that happens all too often. We develop habits for quick food that go against our health goals, and that is why I strongly promote good baseline eating habits and a well-stocked fridge, freezer and pantry with the right foods.

If you eat rice or potatoes at least 3 times every week, this is a staple and part of your baseline. If you have a snack every day and it's the same food item, then it is part of your baseline eating even though it is considered a snack. This is also true for what we drink. If you have a glass of orange juice every day or every other day, then this is part of your baseline. If you have a glass of OJ only on Sunday, then this is not considered part of your baseline. Consider it a treat.

Other benefits to healthy baseline foods are: they allow us to fast for longer periods of time, we don't overeat as often, we won't wake up feeling hungry first thing in the morning, and we won't have to deal with the mid-afternoon bonk.

RECOMMENDED READING

Canton Ketogenic Diet For Cancer, Type I Diabetes & Other Ailments - Elaine Canton

PART VII

ARE YOU READY TO TAKE ON MORE OF A CHALLENGE?

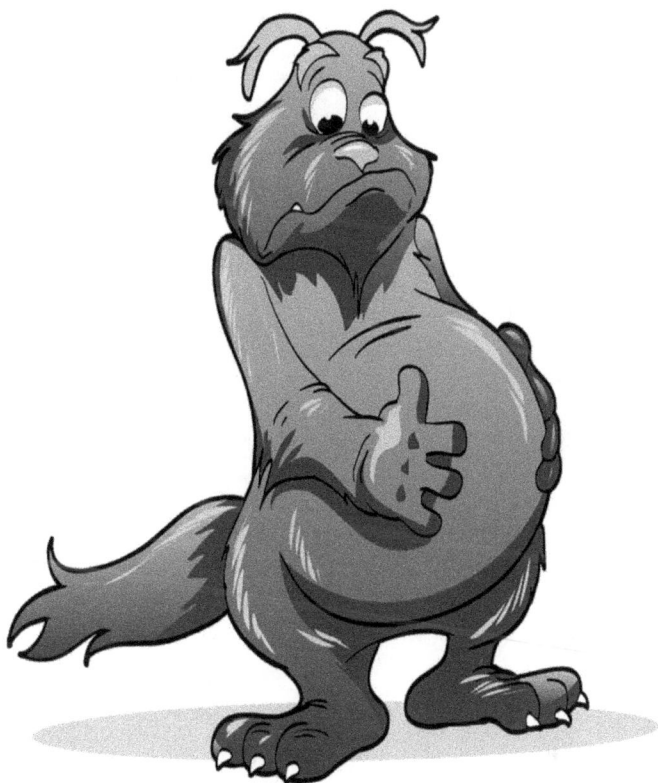

24

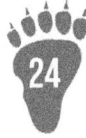

RESTORING YOUR GUT HEALTH

RESTORE YOUR GUT HEALTH

H OW WELL WE output (poop) is an indicator of how healthy our stomach is. The Bristol stool chart below gives us something to refer to when discussing a person's digestion. Ideally we poop at a level 4 most of the time. If not, it can be an indicator our stomach is not in perfect health. Other indicators are constant yeast infections, skin irritations, fatigue, and a sore tummy.

Poor gut flora leads to inflammation; this is one of the root causes of many of today's health problems, including diabetes. Inflammation inhibits fat cells from performing their job properly, making insulin's job even harder in trying to maintain a balance of blood sugar.

Bristol Stool Chart

Type 1		Separate hard lumps, like nuts (hard to pass)
Type 2		Sausage-shaped but lumpy
Type 3		Like a sausage but with cracks on the surface
Type 4		Like a sausage or snake, smooth and soft
Type 5		Soft blobs with clear-cut edges
Type 6		Fluffy pieces with ragged edges, a mushy stool
Type 7		Watery, no solid pieces. **Entirely Liquid**

Many of our modern lifestyles contribute to unhealthy gut flora. These include:

- Taking antibiotics, NSAIDs, and birth control pills.

- A dietary staple of bad and ok carbohydrates.

- Diets low in quality fiber.

- A dietary staple that includes GMO grains: wheat, soy, corn, and sugar.

- A dietary staple including bad fats and products with altered proteins.

- Chronic stress and infections.

Essentially, the healthier our gut, the healthier we are.

. . . .

STEPS TO HELP TO RESTORE YOUR GUT'S HEALTH.

The easy steps:

- Break the vicious cycle of sugar and pro-cessed food addiction, as outlined in chapter 5. This is the key that enables us to stop feeding the bad bacteria in our gut and prevent inflammation from spreading throughout the rest of our body.

- Include more fresh vegetables from the good carbohydrate list, especially green veggies, like kale, spinach, and leafy greens. These will help to balance our body's pH and add extra fiber to our diet.

- Take a probiotic and digestive enzyme daily. We find that Costco brands tend to be good with reasonable prices, or go to a health food store and ask for some advice. Keep in mind that a higher price doesn't mean better quality. When looking for a probiotic supplement, look for ones that have 2 strains, Lactobacillus GG and Bacillus coagulens.

- Fast as outlined earlier; besides the benefits received from resetting, it also helps in healing our tummy.

- Drink plenty of water. Your body is hydrated if your urine is light in color.

- Replace table salt with a quality sea salt, such as Himalayan sea salt or Real Salt. Salt helps our body produce hydrochloric acid which it uses to break down any food we've eaten. Traditional iodized table salt has anticlumping agents which impede our digestion and wreak havoc with our good gut bacteria. Go ahead and throw away all of this type of salt and start using unrefined sea salt today.

The next steps:

- Fiber should be an important staple in everyone's diet; it is actually a probiotic. It helps to slow down how quickly our food digests and feeds the good tummy bacteria. According to Dr. Natashia Campbell who invented the GAPS diet, when a person's gut flora is way out of balance, fiber isn't able to do its job properly and has an opposite effect. If by slowly increasing our daily intake of fiber we experience tummy irritability, this could be a sign our gut flora is way out of balance. I'd recommend reading her book if your gut needs some serious healing.

- Incorporate fermented foods. These are very quick, easy, and inexpensive to make on your own (See our recipe's at www.diabetesmonster.com), or you can find them at a health food store. Fermented vegetables are a great source of probiotics, vitamin K2, and fiber. Eating them a couple times a day with or just prior to a meal will help to restore gut health. If you are taking a vitamin D3 supplement, take it with fermented foods.

- Bone broth from beef, chicken or turkey is another easy item to make and is great for healing our stomach. (See our recipe's online)

- Use coconut oil. It is a superfood full of body-friendly fatty acids that have antimicrobial, antifungal, and antiviral properties. Throw away all vegetable oils, including canola and peanut oil. These are too high in omega-6 fatty acids and do more harm than good. Coconut oil is good for all of your cooking needs, while olive oil is great for salad dressing and any low temperature cooking. I also like to use butter for low temperature cooking.

Supplements

- If you did throw away table salt, you will need to supplement with a product that has both iodine and iodide. I like a product called Ioderol, but others also have the combination of iodine and iodide. Supplement with 2-3 mg per day.

- Take a high quality fish oil sourced from molecularly distilled fish oils as these are naturally high in EPA and DHA. Look for brands that have been independently tested and guaranteed to be free of heavy metals. Take 700-1,000 mg of EPA and 200-500 mg of DHA daily. Fish oil is an omega-3 fatty acid and is a great way to bring our omega-6 to omega-3 ratio back into balance. Omega 3s help in reducing inflammation and support our immune system.

- Zinc: Our bodies use zinc to form digestive enzymes and it is used in regulating hormones (remember insulin and vitamin D are hormones). Take 15 mg per day, up to 30 mg if you are vegetarian or do not eat a lot of animal based foods.

- L-glutamine: This helps to heal and seal the gut and is used by people who have "leaky" gut. L-glutamine helps to synthesize proteins and is important to gluconeogenesis, which helps regulate blood sugars.

Supplement with 5-10 mg total per day and spread it out throughout the day. For instance take 3 mg with 2-3 meals. Start with a low dose and increase to your desired amount.

Herbs

- Cinnamon helps improve digestion and aids in balancing blood sugar levels.

- Other herbs to help relax your GI tract include turmeric, mint, slippery elm, marshmallow root, and deglycyrrhizinated licorice.

. . . .

Do you get severe colds or the flu that seem to last a long time? This can be another sign your stomach health needs work and or that your body has a lot of inflammation.

One of the best ways to help prevent the common cold and influenza is by optimizing our immune system by optimizing our gut health. When we eat sugar or substances like trans fats or artificial sweeteners which are foreign to our bodies, we are asking our body to fight against these extra invaders when our immune system is already working overtime. Having an optimum immune system is absolutely necessary when taking on the good fight to improve our health.

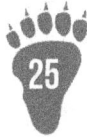

DETERMINE A NORMAL WEIGHT RANGE

THIS STEP MAY take some time, and you may find yourself adjusting your normal weight range as you learn more and as your body changes. The key is to be brutally honest in determining a normal weight. Just because the new normal is people being 10-20 pounds overweight doesn't mean this is what's best for our health. Ten to twenty pounds leads to a much higher risk of diabetes and cardiovascular disease.

One scene from a movie that I really enjoy is in Black Hawk Down. Major General William Garrison radioed Lt. Col. Danny McKnight for a no BS assessment of a situation. McNight was leading the ground forces in Mogadishu, in the middle of a situation which was going from bad to worse. Garrison was at the command center outside the city and needed to know exactly what was going on so he could make an informed decision on how to direct McNight, and to provide the same informed decision making to the other teams scattered around the war torn town.

Having well-informed, accurate and proper information is critical in decision making. In order to determine our normal weight, start with a no BS assessment, including the following ratios:

WAIST-TO-HIP RATIO

This is accomplished by dividing our waist circumference by our hip circumference. The resulting ratio determines if we are in a normal range or above it.

There are a couple of options to measuring our waist and it is easier having someone to help. Stand erect with your arms hanging loosely by your side. Measure at the smallest diameter above your belly button (measure 1" above your belly button if you have an irregular shape). Or suck your stomach in as much as possible and measure right at your belly button. You will likely get two different results; this is ok and it is part of learning what is right for you. Write down your results.

Next, measure the widest area around your buttocks. Divide your waist measurements by the hip measurement. The result is your waist-to-hip ratio.

A normal waist-to-hip ratio for men is below 0.90 and below 0.85 for women.

If your waist-to-hip ratio is above normal, even by as little as 0.01 (0.91 for men and 0.86 for women), this is an indication that your risk of getting diabetes has gone up significantly.

There is no one perfect measurement to tell you what a normal weight should be. Waist-to-hip ratio is not perfect because of the variety of shapes and sizes we have. But it is a strong indicator for the majority of us because we store our fat first in the stomach area. Use your own judgement, but when used with other measurements, the waist-to-hip ratio is, in my opinion, a really good indicator.

WAIST-TO-HEIGHT RATIO

A waist-to-height ratio may be a better ratio for people who are more muscular. This ratio is calculated the same way as the waist-to-hip ratio. Take your waist circumference measurement and divide it by your height in inches. A waist-to-height ratio of less than 0.5 is considered normal.

BMI (BODY MASS INDEX)

I'm not a big fan of BMI mainly because it does not take into consideration how muscular someone is or their body shape. It is simply a tool to help determine if the normal weight you are considering is right. BMI is a number based on height, weight and gender. A normal BMI is between 20 and 25. Below 20 is considered underweight, 25 to 30 is considered overweight, and above 30 is obese. Use the chart on the next page to determine your BMI.

The World Health Organization maintains that a waist size above 37" for men and 31.5" for women means you are at an increased risk of health problems, and above 40" for men and 34.6" for women puts you into a substantially increased risk, regardless of your height.

Body Mass Index (BMI) Charts

http://www.vertex42.com/ExcelTemplates/bmi-chart.html

Vertex42

© 2009 Vertex42 LLC

Body Mass Index (BMI) Table for Adults

Obese (>30) Overweight (25-30) Normal (18.5-25) Underweight (<18.5)

WEIGHT — **HEIGHT in feet/inches and centimeters**

lbs (kg)	4'8"	4'9"	4'10"	4'11"	5'0"	5'1"	5'2"	5'3"	5'4"	5'5"	5'6"	5'7"	5'8"	5'9"	5'10"	5'11"	6'0"	6'1"	6'2"	6'3"	6'4"	6'5"
	142cm	145	147	150	152	155	157	160	163	165	168	170	173	175	178	180	183	185	188	191	193	196
260 (117.9)	58	56	54	53	51	49	48	46	45	43	42	41	40	38	37	36	35	34	33	32	32	31
255 (115.7)	57	55	53	51	50	48	47	45	44	42	41	40	39	38	37	36	35	34	33	32	31	30
250 (113.4)	56	54	52	50	49	47	46	44	43	42	40	39	38	37	36	35	34	33	32	31	30	30
245 (111.1)	55	53	51	49	48	46	45	43	42	41	40	38	37	36	35	34	33	32	31	31	30	29
240 (108.9)	54	52	50	48	47	45	44	43	41	40	39	38	36	35	34	33	33	32	31	30	29	28
235 (106.6)	53	51	49	47	46	44	43	42	40	39	38	37	36	35	34	33	32	31	30	29	29	28
230 (104.3)	52	50	48	46	45	43	42	41	39	38	37	36	35	34	33	32	31	30	30	29	28	27
225 (102.1)	50	49	47	45	44	43	41	40	39	37	36	35	34	33	32	31	31	30	29	28	27	27
220 (99.8)	49	48	46	44	43	42	40	39	38	37	36	34	33	32	32	31	30	29	28	27	27	26
215 (97.5)	48	47	45	43	42	41	39	38	37	36	35	34	33	32	31	30	29	28	28	27	26	25
210 (95.3)	47	45	44	42	41	40	38	37	36	35	34	33	32	31	30	29	28	28	27	26	26	25
205 (93.0)	46	44	43	41	40	39	37	36	35	34	33	32	31	30	29	29	28	27	26	26	25	24
200 (90.7)	45	43	42	40	39	38	37	35	34	33	32	31	30	30	29	28	27	26	26	25	24	24
195 (88.5)	44	42	41	39	38	37	36	35	33	32	31	31	30	29	28	27	26	26	25	24	24	23
190 (86.2)	43	41	40	38	37	36	35	34	33	32	31	30	29	28	27	26	26	25	24	24	23	23
185 (83.9)	41	40	39	37	36	35	34	33	32	31	30	29	28	27	27	26	25	24	24	23	23	22
180 (81.6)	40	39	38	36	35	34	33	32	31	30	29	28	27	27	26	25	24	24	23	22	22	21
175 (79.4)	39	38	37	35	34	33	32	31	30	29	28	27	27	26	25	24	24	23	22	22	21	21
170 (77.1)	38	37	36	34	33	32	31	30	29	28	27	27	26	25	24	24	23	22	22	21	21	20
165 (74.8)	37	36	34	33	32	31	30	29	28	27	27	26	25	24	24	23	22	22	21	21	20	20
160 (72.6)	36	35	33	32	31	30	29	28	27	27	26	25	24	24	23	22	22	21	21	20	19	19
155 (70.3)	35	34	32	31	30	29	28	27	27	26	25	24	24	23	22	22	21	20	20	19	19	18
150 (68.0)	34	32	31	30	29	28	27	27	26	25	24	23	23	22	22	21	20	20	19	19	18	18
145 (65.8)	33	31	30	29	28	27	27	26	25	24	23	23	22	21	21	20	20	19	19	18	18	17
140 (63.5)	31	30	29	28	27	26	26	25	24	23	23	22	21	21	20	20	19	18	18	17	17	17
135 (61.2)	30	29	28	27	26	26	25	24	23	22	22	21	21	20	19	19	18	18	17	17	16	16
130 (59.0)	29	28	27	26	25	25	24	23	22	22	21	20	20	19	19	18	18	17	17	16	16	15
125 (56.7)	28	27	26	25	24	24	23	22	21	21	20	20	19	18	18	17	17	16	16	16	15	15
120 (54.4)	27	26	25	24	23	23	22	21	21	20	19	19	18	18	17	17	16	16	15	15	15	14
115 (52.2)	26	25	24	23	22	22	21	20	20	19	19	18	17	17	16	16	16	15	15	14	14	14
110 (49.9)	25	24	23	22	21	21	20	19	19	18	18	17	17	16	16	15	15	15	14	14	13	13
105 (47.6)	24	23	22	21	21	20	19	19	18	17	17	16	16	16	15	15	14	14	13	13	13	12
100 (45.4)	22	22	21	20	20	19	18	18	17	17	16	16	15	15	14	14	14	13	13	12	12	12
95 (43.1)	21	21	20	19	19	18	17	17	16	16	15	15	14	14	14	13	13	13	12	12	12	11
90 (40.8)	20	19	19	18	18	17	16	16	15	15	15	14	14	13	13	13	12	12	12	11	11	11
85 (38.6)	19	18	18	17	17	16	16	15	15	14	14	13	13	13	12	12	12	11	11	11	10	10
80 (36.3)	18	17	17	16	16	15	15	14	14	13	13	13	12	12	11	11	11	11	10	10	10	9

Note: BMI values rounded to the nearest whole number. BMI categories based on CDC (Centers for Disease Control and Prevention) criteria.

www.vertex42.com

BMI = Weight[kg] / (Height[m] x Height[m]) = 703 x Weight[lb] / (Height[in] x Height[in])

© 2009 Vertex42 LLC

BMI Chart created by Vertex42.com. Used with permission.

Another good measurement is the 9 point body fat measurement. This tells us our % of body fat. The problem is we need calipers for measuring, and someone to perform the test. Some gyms or health practitioners will offer this measurement as a service. The bonus to going to one of these places is they are used to taking the measurements and we are likely to get a more accurate measurement.

If you get this measurement done, compare your results to charts you can find online for what your body fat % should be based on your age, height, and body type.

. . . .

Next is to put your measurements together to determine a good weight range. This is the point where you should be very honest and as realistic as possible. Take your best shot at a reasonable weight then weigh daily as outlined in the easy steps in order to monitor your progress.

BODY MEASUREMENT CHART

	Target range	Actual	Within range?
Sucked in waist measurement	---		---
Stand erect waist measurement	---		---
Hip measurement	---		---
Height measurement	---		---
Waist to Hip Rasio	Male < 0.90 Female < 0.85		
BMI	18.5 – 24.9		
Waist to Height Ratio	< 0.50		

Be prepared to alter an ideal range as you learn more about what a normal healthy weight should be. If you have made some serious dietary changes by cutting out bad and ok carbohydrates, by not drinking calories, or in how frequently and intense you exercise, you will likely find your body changing. It's ok to change what your normal weight range is. Just make sure you are adjusting this range for the right reasons.

In the table above, if you answered no to "Within range?" on any of the measurements, then you are likely not within a normal healthy range and should consider changes to your eating and or exercising habits to allow your body to get within a normal healthy range. The only exception I would make to this is if you are within range on waist-to-hip and also within range on waist-to-height but slightly high on BMI, as this could be a result of your body type.

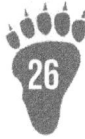

CHOLESTEROL RATIOS

DO YOU KNOW YOUR CHOLESTEROL RATIOS?

COMMON KNOWLEDGE IS that cholesterol seems to come in two flavors, good and bad, or HDL as the good and LDL as the bad. Recent research, according to Dr. Lustig, shows a third cholesterol called VLDL is the bad culprit when it comes to inflammation and cardiovascular disease.

VLDL stands for very low density lipoprotein. This cholesterol is a small enough molecule that it can imbed itself in the lining of our arteries. When too many get trapped it causes blood flow to be restricted and our blood pressure increases. The normal LDL cholesterol molecule is too large to do this; it simply circulates around for use when needed. Not a lot is known of LDL but it appears to be not as bad as has been thought.

According to Dr. Lustig, VLDL is made by your liver

when too much fructose is present. Your liver can only metabolize a small amount of fructose into non-harmful substances, but when it gets overloaded, it turns fructose into a byproduct of triglycerides. Avoiding products such as high fructose corn syrup and agave nectar is very important. Agave nectar is touted as diabetic-friendly because it doesn't have as much glucose so it doesn't raise your blood sugar levels as high as might otherwise be the case, but what it does have is higher amounts of fructose which according to Dr. Lustig is far more damaging.

Have your VLDL checked yearly. You may have to ask specifically for it to be measured as the standard cholesterol panel does not measure it.

Triglycerides is one of the key markers for metabolic syndrome, a level above 150 means you are at risk of serious health issues.

The worst possible combination is if your level of triglycerides is high and you have low amounts of HDL. This is an indication of being at risk for a heart attack and why it is important to get VLDL measured. Discuss this with your doctor immediately, and if they are not up to speed on VLDL then ask them questions about it, even point your doctor to Dr. Lustig's book.

Here are a few recognized formulae for determining optimum cholesterol levels.

1. HDL to Total Cholesterol: Divide your HDL level by your total cholesterol, (HDL + LDL). A normal range is above 24 percent, and ideally it should be above 30 percent.

A ratio below 24 percent means it's time to change your baseline foods and take on more of the easy steps outlined earlier. Levels below 10 percent are considered very dangerous and usually indicate an imminent cardiovascular problem.

2. Triglyceride to HDL: Divide your triglyceride number by your HDL. This ratio should be below 2. Numbers above 2 indicate possible insulin-resistance and intervention as outlined throughout is required to avoid health risks.

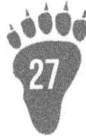

ALTERNATIVE AND ARTIFICIAL SWEETENERS

ALTERNATIVE AND ARTIFICIAL SWEETENERS, GOOD OR BAD?

DO YOU KNOW someone who's tried to break a diet soda habit? It seems almost impossible and requires a few days of withdrawal. Even when someone gets past this point, the recidivism rate, or the number who go back to drinking diet soda is very high.

If zero calorie sweeteners were a key to weight loss, wouldn't more people be closer to their normal weight? Researchers have now unlocked why this isn't true, and why diabetics should stay clear of the big 5 artificial sweeteners which are the only ones the FDA has on the GRAS list (Generally Recognized as Safe): saccharin (Sweet 'N Low, Sweet and Low, Sweet Twin, Nectra Sweet); aspartame (Nutrasweet, Equal, Sugar Twin); sucralose

(Splenda); acesulfame, also known as acesulfame potassium (Sunett, Sweet One); and neotame (chemically most like aspartame, and much sweeter than sucrose).

Leptin is a hormone which regulates our appetite. It relies mainly on fibers in natural foods for a signal that we've eaten something and is one of the keys to not overeating. When we consume an artificial sweetener from a soft drink, our brain releases dopamine which activates our pleasure or reward center. Our body is getting mixed messages, pleasure from food but with no calories and no fiber present, leptin has no signal that we have just eaten or drank something. As the effect from the dopamine wears off, our body wants to get back the pleasure feeling which is why we crave fast acting carbohydrates. They are a quick fix to the mixed message. Artificial sweeteners simply do not work for weight loss. In fact they have the opposite effect.

Diabetics should stay completely clear of these nasty chemical-laden artificial sweeteners because the last thing you need is a signal to eat fast acting carbohydrates which worsen your condition. Researchers have found artificial sweeteners alter your metabolic pathways associated with metabolic disease and that aspartame actually worsens insulin-sensitivity more than sugar. Both of these are at the core of diabetes and are further reasons to completely avoid anything with artificial sweeteners.

Research has also proven artificial sweeteners disrupts our gut flora, raising our risk of obesity and diabetes. Gut flora as you've learned is a key to a healthy life.

If you are looking for more evidence, I'd recommend

researching for yourself, but don't go by what a marketer says about their product, or a catchy ad. Research people, like Dr. Peeke. I recommend reading her book, The Hunger Fix.

As of the writing of this book, the only sweetener I'd recommend is actually a dietary supplement called stevia.

Stevia comes from the stevia plant, and I recommend buying a stevia product that has only one ingredient, stevia. Many Stevia producers add fillers, like dextrose or maltodextrin, to make the stevia seem more like sugar, where a teaspoon of their stevia product would be similar to a teaspoon of sugar. But dextrose and maltodextrin are known to cause irritability in your tummy and disrupt your gut flora, so these are best avoided.

Marketers are catching on to stevia's popularity and adding it to their products, but remember marketers are masters of deception. Fortunately what they can't deceive is the ingredients list—and this is why it is so important to always read the list of ingredients.

RECOMMENDED READING

Brain Maker - Dr. David Perlmutter
The Great Cholesterol Con - Anthony Colpo

PART VIII

ALL ABOUT FOOD

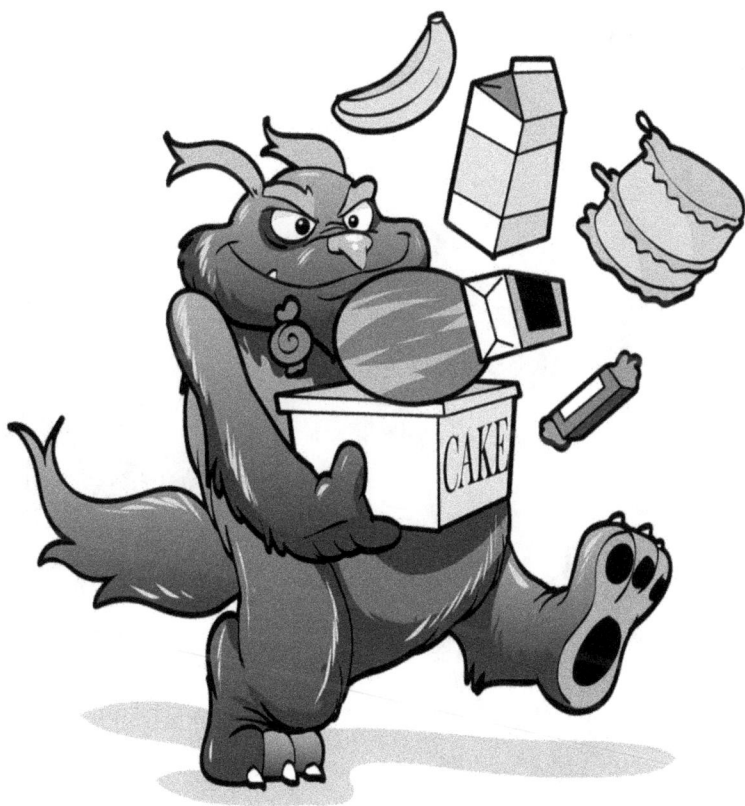

28

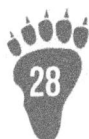

LEARN ABOUT FOODS

QUITE POSSIBLY, THE biggest problem we have with food today is how highly processed it can be. In many instances, the product today is nothing like the original that has been consumed for centuries.

Milk is a good example. It goes through a heating process (pasteurization) that kills the lactase which is the enzyme our bodies use to break down the lactose (sugar). This is one of the reasons why so many people of our generation are lactose-intolerant. Milk is also homogenized to break down the protein into smaller molecules to keep the cream from separating. These smaller protein molecules can cause distress in your intestines.

Most of the natural minerals and vitamins in milk are killed off during these processes. Manufacturers infuse the milk with man-made calcium and vitamin D, which is not nearly as absorbable as the natural ones.

Some states allow the sale of raw milk—milk that has not been pasteurized or homogenized. This is a personal decision whether or not to drink this type of milk. Please do your own research before deciding what is best.

Many grains have had their natural state altered. Wheat is nothing like it was 100 years ago. Today's wheat has a much higher protein content because protein is the most valuable part of the plant. Not surprising that researchers have found a way to alter grains to have higher concentrations of protein.

Eating the entire whole grain may be beneficial on occasion due to the fiber content and minerals, although I still classify them as ok carbohydrates.

Processed versions of grains should be completely avoided. Grains are extruded to make all of the different shapes and sizes of cereals. The extrusion process breaks down the protein molecule into smaller chunks and researchers are finding these smaller proteins lead to poor gut flora. Ninety-nine percent (99%) of all cereals use extruded grains. If you have tummy issues, or you have a child who does, then consider removing all breads and cereals from their diet.

. . . .

The following are some thoughts on popular food items:

EGGS

Eggs are a good source of protein. They contain lutein, vitamin D, all nine essential amino acids, and choline. Our bodies use choline for cell structure and turn it into acetylcholine which is a neurotransmitter required to maintain optimal brain health. Eggs have been part of diets for as long as we know and I'm glad the myth that "eggs are bad" has been debunked.

The source of eggs ranges from mass-produced eggs in over-populated hen farms (CAFOs), to organically-raised free-range chickens. Prices vary but a typical organic-fed chicken egg costs about 40 cents per egg. That's 80 cents for a great snack of 2 eggs and a heck of a lot cheaper than the processed grain bars disguised as natural all healthy protein bars.

Farmers' markets are a great place to find eggs. They make for a great second breakfast or snack because they have lots of good fat and protein which will keep your hunger under control much more so than a carbohydrate snack.

BUTTER

We have been through an era where eating margarine and other butter substitutes were thought to be healthier than butter. There are many who still believe this, especially when marketers tag their products as heart-friendly. Research has clearly proven that these trans-fat-laden products are anything but healthy and should be completely avoided.

The real issue with butter is the source. Most butter in grocery stores today comes from a CAFO where the milk cows are injected with antibiotics and or growth hormones. This is the real reason to avoid butter. Try to find organic butter and ideally find a source where the cows are grass fed and free of antibiotics and growth hormones.

OILS

The best oil to use for cooking is coconut oil because it does not break down at high heat. It has medium chain fatty acids that your body uses to function properly and is anti-fungal and anti-bacterial.

Olive oil and avocado oil are excellent for salad dressings. These oils are monounsaturated fats high in omega-3s. Body-friendly fats like olive and avocado oil may have a positive effect on your cholesterol levels, help normalize blood clotting, and may be beneficial in your body's ability to control blood sugar and insulin levels.

There are no health benefits to any of the other oils (peanut oil, soybean oil, safflower, canola, and the like)— only health risks. Removing all of those oils from your house right now could be one of the healthiest things you ever do.

SALT

Regular table salt is highly processed to remove all trace minerals. It is processed down to two ingredients, sodium (Na) and chlorine (Cl). An additive is used to keep the salt from clumping. This additive is known to cause irritation in the tummy that can lead to poor gut flora. The benefit to regular table salt is iodine is added, but this is not a good enough reason to use table salt.

A better salt is Celtic sea salt, Himalayan sea salt or a product from the salt beds of Utah known as Real Salt. These are typically unrefined salts that have trace metals and minerals that absorb into your body better because they are unrefined. The only downside to these salts is they do not have iodine and our bodies need iodine.

You can get iodine from eating yogurt, eggs, strawberries, cheese, seaweed, kelp, kale, broccoli, cabbage, peanuts, Brussels sprouts, turnips and kohlrabi. There are many iodine supplements on the market and the best have both iodine and iodide.

OATMEAL

A staple for many in North American is to have oatmeal for breakfast. Oatmeal is marketed as heart healthy and good for us because it has dietary fiber, protein, fat and many vitamins and minerals. The problem with oatmeal is it is mainly a carbohydrate and the fats it contains are almost all omega-6. This makes it anything but heart healthy.

The glycemic index of oatmeal is 55, which means it takes a few minutes longer to digest than a bagel with a glycemic index of 90—but it is merely minutes. It still metabolizes quickly and will spike your body's insulin level and that is before adding fruit, sugar, and or syrup.

Packaged or minute oatmeal is a highly processed food to be avoided. As in most processed foods, the fiber has been removed for it to be cooked quicker, not to mention all of the other added ingredients.

If giving up oatmeal is simply too much, try to make it healthier. Cook half as much oatmeal and add in some raw nuts and seeds. An example would be to add raw chia seeds, flax seeds, hemp hearts, and macadamia nuts. If you need to sweeten it, use stevia or if you are not eating oatmeal as a staple, then try sweetening with local raw honey.

I list oatmeal as an ok carbohydrate, but only oatmeal that is the whole grain. Packaged oatmeal is definitely "bad." If you are healing, then completely avoid oatmeal until your metabolic syndrome markers are back to normal.

PROTEIN

Proteins come from animals, fish, vegetables or plants and each has its own benefits. Animal and fish protein are high in saturated fats, omega-3 essential fatty acids and typically have the highest amount of protein by density. Vegetable and plant proteins come with other very good benefits such as fiber, vitamins and minerals.

Our bodies do not produce CLA (conjugated linoleic acid). We need to get it through what we eat and grass-fed beef is one of the best sources. CLA helps our bodies fight cancer, asthma, high blood pressure, inflammation, cardiovascular disease and is known to help improve insulin-resistance along with providing our bodies with high quality minerals like iron, zinc and B vitamins.

I was surprised to find that cows that are either raised in a CAFO, or are grain-finished, do not produce CLA. It is a physiological change that happens when they eat corn and grain. Why then are cows fed corn and grain? The answer is because it fattens them up quicker, and it's a cheaper way to feed them. It is now about profits and feeding the masses, not what is best.

Maybe even worse is that CAFO cows are routinely fed antibiotics to overcome their unhealthy living conditions, and growth hormones to maximize profits from each cow. Almost all beef in stores is from a CAFO. Do your best to avoid it. Look for organic beef, or beef raised without antibiotics and hormones. If you routinely eat beef and have some freezer space, consider purchasing beef in larger quantities from a local grass-fed beef producer.

Avoid generic dairy products for the same reasons. Look for products which state the source of their milk, or that no antibiotics or growth hormones are used. When you find good sources of dairy, eat the full fat versions to get as much CLA as possible. I know this is contrary to what most people believe, but good dairy products are some of the best body-friendly fats you can get. Just remember if you are adding in more of these body-friendly fats, you need to cut down on your intake of bad and ok carbohydrates.

When looking for other animal protein, such as pork, chicken and turkey, look for animals which are free of anti-biotics and growth hormones. Read the package. If the company is promoting how healthy they raise their animals, then they are likely a very good source. It is best to assume any chicken, beef and pork in grocery stores is CAFO-raised unless the package states otherwise. If this is what your budget allows, then try to eat the leanest cuts and do not eat the fat, but I would encourage you to avoid any CAFO products.

Seafood can also be very nutritious and healthy. Whenever possible, eat only wild seafood, such as wild salmon. As of the writing of this book, farmed-seafood should be eaten infrequently, if at all. Farm-raised seafood is both ecologically unfriendly, and potentially a health risk if too much is consumed.

Another caution is in how much shell fish you eat. Recent studies show that muscles and scallops have higher amounts of mercury, but they also have very good nutri-tional value, eat them in moderation.

What about when you go to a restaurant? You have to decide for yourself how far to take it. For instance, I will order a steak now and then at a restaurant knowing it is likely from a CAFO. I enjoy the meal and will not eat the fat; however, rarely will I eat salmon unless I know it has been wild-caught.

Legumes are another source of protein, although they also come with plenty of carbohydrates. This is why I have them listed as an ok carbohydrate. If you are healing, then avoid all legumes until you get back to good, then treat them as an ok carbohydrate as I've outlined.

CHEESE

One of my go-to snacks is cheese. I only buy cheese where I know the source of the milk. Cheese is a great snack because it is full of body-friendly fats, healthy protein, plus a few good carbohydrates. This is another of those myths to get past—that cheese causes heart disease. Just don't eat your cheese with a cracker; learn to enjoy a piece of cheese as is, or put it on a slice of cucumber.

One of the defining research papers on nutrition in the 1960s involved Scandinavian fishermen. The researcher, Ancel Keys, wanted to prove that fats were bad. He cited that these Scandinavian fishermen who ate multiple sandwiches each day with thick cuts of cheese had a higher incidence of heart disease because of the amount of saturated fat they were eating from the cheese. What he failed to mention was along with the two large pieces of bread that made the sandwich, the fishermen also drank a few beers. So was it the cheese? Or now that we know about what causes insulin-resistance, was it the bread and beer? I put my money on the latter.

PRODUCE

A key question is if we should use organic produce versus non-organic. The easy answer to this is yes, it is worth it whenever possible. Buying fresh organic produce, however, may not be that easy. It does cost more which can be prohibitive and it is not always available. Here is a well-publicized list of the clean 15. This produce is ok to buy as non-organic. The dirty dozen is produce to be avoided unless you can find them as organic.

Clean 15	Dirty Dozen
Avocados	Apples
Sweet corn	Strawberries
Pineapples	Grapes
Cabbage	Nectarines (imported)
Sweet peas (frozen)	Peaches
Sweet potatoes	Spinach
Cantaloupe (domestic)	Snap peas (imported)
Onions	Sweet bell peppers
Asparagus	Cucumbers
Mangoes	Cherry tomatoes
Papayas	Celery
Kiwi	Potatoes
Eggplant	
Grapefruit	caution
Cauliflower	Hot Peppers
	Blueberries

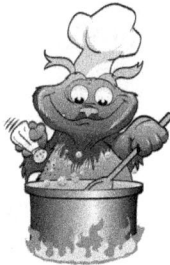

Learning to store fresh produce is just as important as selecting it. Someone in the produce department of the grocery store or the produce manager would have some good insight into how to do this. Vegetables, like leafy greens, celery, beans, and carrots, need to be stored in the fridge in plastic bags so they don't wilt. Other items such as tomatoes and citrus fruit maintain their best flavor if stored at room temperature. Keep tomatoes in the light on the counter, but citrus will keep longer in the dark. If you need to extend the shelf-life of either of these, then move them to the refrigerator. Some fruits, like cucumbers, should be stored in the vegetable drawer in your fridge without a bag. Don't store them with apples or tomatoes as they hasten the ripening process. There are quite a few do's and don'ts like this but you will learn over time what works. Don't let all these "rules" stop you from buying produce. They are just guidelines to prolong the shelf life to help you avoid throwing out more produce because it's gone bad.

It is very important to wash produce prior to using it, and this goes for organic and non-organic produce. Rinsing under cold flowing water will remove dirt, pesticides, and anything else that may have been sprayed on the produce to maintain it during shipment to the market. The produce needs to be dried completely before storing it. Salad spinners are great for removing water from leafy greens and small vegetables. A rule of thumb is that it is ok to pre-wash vegetables that are going to be stored in the fridge. However, only wash vegetables room temperature vegetables as you use them.

Growing your own vegetables can be a fun experience for some. This can range from an outside garden, to growing microgreens inside. Microgreens are easy to grow and are packed full of nutrition. These are a great way to start gardening. (See how to grow microgreens at our website)

WATER

Water has become another of those slightly controversial subjects which may sound a bit crazy. Most everyone agrees that we should all drink water, although too much water may lead to mineral depletion. Having up to 8 glasses a day should keep our bodies hydrated and our cells satisfied.

The controversy is what type of water. Until the advent of indoor plumbing and running water, we drank water from streams, springs, lakes and ponds. A problem with running water in our houses today is it is not the same as water from streams and springs. It has been filtered, stripping of many of its minerals. Chemicals, like chlorine, bromine, and or fluorine, have been added and our bodies are not meant to digest these. Research is linking many health problems to these foreign chemicals.

The downside to drinking bottled water or RO (reverse osmosis) water is they too are depleted of minerals, but we can supplement for the minerals and electrolytes by eating a healthy diet of meat, vegetables, nuts and seeds.

ALTERNATIVE MILKS

Alternative milks come in different varieties: original, unsweetened, vanilla, etc. What I couldn't believe the first time I saw these was the original variety was actually sweetened with sugar. It has six grams of sugar per one cup serving. That is the same as adding two sugar cubes to that one cup serving. The only variety which has zero sugars are the unsweetened ones. Be careful when buying these milks! I can't wait to see the day when original means "no sugar."

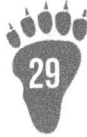

29

MEALS AND SHOPPING

BASELINE MEALS

Breakfast:

THIS IS THE meal we use to break our overnight fast. Somewhere along the way, we have lost the intent of breakfast. Marketers would have us believe we need something to kick-start our day, and we should eat their product because it gets us going. Well, guess what—good carbohydrates, healthy protein and body-friendly fats also get us going, and they keep us going longer without spiking insulin. Our body just spent the past number of hours resetting itself—don't assault it with a poor breakfast choice.

Because of the stresses of work, school, children, and others, breakfast has turned into a, "what can I eat quickly" meal. However, it should not be about cereal and toast because they are all bad carbohydrates which spike insulin and sets us up for feelings of hunger and cravings for carbohydrates all day long. Where is it written in our genetic code to eat these fast-acting carbohydrates for breakfast? It isn't, although marketers would have you believe it is. Breakfast should be about fueling our body for whatever we are going to do in the morning. A quick breakfast could simply be eating leftovers from the night before; why not, they are ready to eat.

Many people have turned to smoothies for breakfast which I believe is a good thing, as long as you are mindful of the ingredients and don't use a lot of fruit. For some reason, most powders are called protein-powder because their original target was body builders who were looking to boost their protein intake in order to become more muscular. If you are using a powder, read the ingredients. Are there any chemical names in it? Is it high in protein and carbohydrates? If it is a flavored powder, are the sweeteners sugar and/or artificial sweeteners? There are very few protein powders which I would recommend, especially if you use them as a staple. The protein itself should either be plant-based, like an organic pea protein, or whey concentrate if it is from a good source like grass-fed beef. Avoid all whey isolate because the protein has been altered. As I've stated many times throughout, researchers are linking all altered proteins to intestinal inflammation. Remember this is a staple in your diet so do the work to find a product that uses unaltered ingredients.

Eggs are a great breakfast item because they are high in protein, body-friendly fats and can be made quickly. If you are making an omelet, cut the ingredients the night before if time is at a premium in the morning.

Here is a quick breakfast option: Cut a few slices of cucumber onto a plate while you fry a couple of eggs. Add a thin slice of cheese on top of the egg towards the end. Put the egg onto the cucumber, sprinkle a little paprika or chili powder on top, salt and pepper, and voila—a quick hearty breakfast.

It's ok to add bacon or sausage once in a while as long as they are nitrate-free. In fact, only eat processed meats that are free of nitrates and low in sodium.

If you are going to eat oatmeal, then make sure it is healthier oatmeal as I've described and try to not eat it every morning.

Getting your mind right about wanting to eat a healthier breakfast is the first step; then learn to be creative. Choose foods from the good carbohydrate list, healthy proteins and body-friendly fats.

Lunch & Dinner

These meals should include a healthy protein, vegetables and salad. If you are going to eat something from the ok carbohydrate list, try to have it in an earlier meal. Eating these types of carbohydrates later in the day will make it harder to make it through to bedtime without wanting to snack.

As in my story while meeting with my attorney, make good choices if you end up at a salad bar. Don't go for the baked potato. Instead, go for a protein, vegetables and a salad and eat lots of veggies. These are the carbohydrates your body knows what to do with.

Sandwiches seem to be a preferred lunch item. Instead of bread, use large lettuce leaves or cut a pepper in half and use it instead of bread. When using lettuce, it may be best to take the ingredients separately and put it together when you are ready to eat.

Pasta is another staple that has crept into people's lives. The noodles themselves are really just a carrier for the sauce, but they are all bad carbohydrates. Even the ones marketed as being healthy, all natural, organic, whole grain, etc., are all bad carbohydrates. Alternatives to pasta are spaghetti squash and zucchini. The zucchini pasta recipe on our website is about as easy as pasta can be. Even easier than boiling water. With zucchini pasta you are eating 4 grams of carbohydrates versus 43 grams in even the best whole wheat, natural organic pasta.

Another key if you are healing is to avoid overeating at dinner time. You may want to eat a lot thinking this meal needs to sustain you through a 12-hour fasting goal, but overeating simply sets you up to want to eat more. Overeating causes the hormones I've described throughout this book to be unable to do their job as effectively.

. . . .

See www.diabetesmonster.com for a complete list of foods by carbohydrate category.

. . . .

SHOPPING

One of the keys to making quick and easy meals is the time and thoughtfulness we put into shopping and what we have on hand in the pantry, fridge and/or freezer. Going back to chapter 2 and getting your mind right also applies to shopping and cooking. Once we appreciate how important it is, learning will become much easier. If you think it is a chore, odds are you will continue to struggle with this part of healing and being healthy.

Our shopping culture in North America is so different than in Europe. Europeans will shop for their produce, vegetables and meat almost every day but they have convenient local markets. In North America, shopping has become more centralized and usually requires a planned outing, so take time to plan your outing. There are endless possibilities for making lists, from smart phones to paper, just get in the habit of making a list when you think through your meals.

Keep shopping simple. I've taught a number of people to fly fish which requires some basic casting skills. The best place to practice casting is at a park and not when you are out fishing where you are focused on the fish. Once you have the basics of casting down, catching fish becomes easier because you can cast more easily to where the fish are. Your skills will continue to improve each time you fish. The same is true with shopping. Start by learning what you and the others who you are buying for like, and as long as it is part of your eating plan then go with your list and stick to it. As you get more comfortable with your eating plan you can learn to experiment with other items at the store.

A few thoughts on shopping:

- Try to avoid shopping when you are hungry, or if this is not an option, stick to your list and be quick.

- Avoid all packaged products unless you are happy with their ingredients. Don't fool yourself; if you don't know what an ingredient is, your body probably doesn't know what it is either.

- Farmers' markets can be a great source of locally grown produce and meats. Not all are organic, but by getting to know the farmer, you know how they tend their animals and crops.

- Try to remember the "dirty dozen" when buying produce and either buy organic or avoid these items.

- Cook extra food when time allows and freeze it for quick leftover meals. These should be far healthier than any pre-packaged food from the store.

- Become a master of the stir-fry. Experiment with sauces, marinating meat, and so forth, and don't overcook your vegetables.

- Gadgets can make cooking a lot of fun and make preparation a lot quicker.

- Join online ketogenic, paleo or low-carb recipe sharing sites.

- Learn from others and don't be afraid to ask for help.

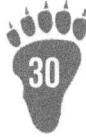

30

EMERGENCY FOODS & SNACKS

EMERGENCY FOODS

SOME OF THE best emergency foods are leftovers from meals you've prepared. Freeze the extra's if you aren't going to eat them in the next day or two.

Other good emergency foods to have on hand are canned tuna and salmon. When purchasing canned items, ensure the ingredients include just tuna or salmon. If the tuna is packed in a light oil, ensure it is packed in olive oil. The caution here is that these canned foods can be high in sodium depending on their ingredients, so if you're like me and have reached that magic age of presbyopia, put on your glasses and read the label.

A caution on tuna is that it contains higher amounts of mercury, so don't make it a staple. Canned tuna is great as emergency food or as a planned meal once and a while.

Other good emergency foods are nuts and seeds which can be combined into a granola (preferably grainless). Chia seeds, flax seeds and hemp seeds are high in protein, high in omega-3 essential fatty acids and overall good for you. You can combine these with some nuts then add to yogurt, or to fruit to make a perfect cereal. If you add unsweetened coconut or almond milk, you will keep the total sugar count down. You can add a protein powder, favorite liquid and or yogurt to these nuts and seeds which makes a healthy and sustaining smoothie.

The next step is learning to sprout and dehydrate your nuts and seeds. Sprouting releases enzymes in the seed that make them easier to digest. Soaking nuts removes tannins which cause tummy irritability. Dehydrate at less than one hundred and ten degrees Fahrenheit to keep the food alive.

More good foods to have on hand are cheese and nut butters. Cheese is an excellent source of protein and minerals, but read the label on the cheese. Cheese should be in the form of a brick, and not from a can. A lot of the highly marketed cheeses have additives and sugar that take what could be a good snack and make it harmful to your body. Finding cheese from organically raised cows that is free of antibiotics and growth hormones is always best. Goat cheese is another very good option, that is, if you don't mind the taste of goat's milk.

Ground almond butter or other nut butters are also great for snacks as long as you don't put them onto a cracker. These can be spread on apples or celery as a quick snack, or simply have a spoonful. You may want to check at a local health food store as a lot of them will grind fresh almonds or other nuts right there for you. This way you can get the grind level you like, and it ensures freshness. If I haven't mentioned reading the labels enough, I need to mention it again. You want nut butters which are only the ground nut itself. So many of the popular varieties are made with trans fats and sugar.

. . . .

I hope I've convinced you to be a label reader. Next is to learn what some of the fancy words mean, like natural flavors. This can and typically does mean a form of MSG (mono sodium glutamate). These "natural flavors" are used as flavor enhancers but have no nutritional value at all, even worse they are cause severe tummy issues and lead to inflammation. The term "natural flavors" was allowed for companies to be able to hide the ingredients in their secret recipes.

Unfortunately the word "natural" in the food industry really has no meaning. You'd think it would mean: an unaltered ingredient from the earth, sadly it doesn't. If a product says natural, it really doesn't mean anything until you've read the list of ingredients. Remember, if the list of ingredients has some chemical names and not just ingredients from Mother Nature, be careful!

SNACKS

Here are some examples of good snack foods, for those times when you get the munchies:

- Cut vegetables, like carrots, celery, broccoli, cauliflower and others (store in a container of water in the fridge).

- Fresh ground almond butter; have up to a tablespoon at a time up to a couple per day. Spread it on a celery stick or a cucumber slice for some variety or simply eat a spoonful.

- Leftover protein from a meal, such as a piece of chicken, salmon, and so on.

- Nuts and seeds. If possible get raw nuts and seeds as most mixes on the market have some form of bad fat.

  - Good nuts include: almonds, cashews, macadamia, walnuts and pistachios. Avoid too many peanuts as they are actually a legume and are high in total carbohydrates.

  - Good seeds include: sunflower seeds, pumpkin seeds, flax seeds, chia seeds, and hemp seeds.

- Cheese (preferably from grass-fed beef)— have a couple of slices per day

RECIPES

Visit our website for a variety of quick and easy meals. www.diabetesmonster.com

RECOMMENDED READING

Nourishing Traditions - Sally Fallon
The Inflammation Cure - Dr. William Joel Meggs

ACKNOWLEDGMENTS
AND REFERENCES

'D LIKE TO pass along a big thanks to all of those who took time to help me complete the writing of this book, including thoughts on content, grammar and layout. There are too many of you to mention, but you know who you are, "thank you".

Thanks to Dr. Azalia Martinez and Dr. Jon Paul Navar for believing enough in me and my approach to diabetes to write an endorsement for the book cover. Thanks to the late Dr. Paul Navar for leading a revolution towards healthy living, my hope is that this book is in some small way a continuation of the dedicated work he started.

Special thanks to my Dad. I hope I don't come across as being too harsh as I use him in a lot of examples throughout. Unfortunately the people helping him at the time did not have the knowledge or skills to actually help him with his diabetes. I don't believe they intended to be misguiding but they just went along with the standard of care at the time. Unfortunately this standard has not kept up with advancements in research.

It's been seventeen years since my father succumbed to the complications of diabetes. I loved my father and enjoyed being around him. Having him healthy for the last ten years of his life would have been so much easier for him, and my Mom. Plus, I would have loved to have him around for an extra ten to fifteen years. Damn diabetes!

Thanks to my Mom. She taught me to take responsibility for my actions, to never let someone else's words bring me down or to get in the way of what I want to achieve. She has been a great role model for being active and living life.

My children, Kyla and Jordan, along with their families have been great supporters of all of my crazy ideas. I am so fortunate to be close to my children despite the miles that separate us.

Special thanks too to my best friend and very significant other Marsha Navar. Her nutritional guidance and insight are incorporated throughout this book. She is one of the best researchers I've known and I've hired and managed a lot of PhD's throughout my career. Marsha really does walk her talk. She also has an incredible cooking talent, lucky me! Her recipe's, which are perfect for anyone concerned with Diabetes (and Celiac's) can be found on our website (www.diabetesmonster.com).

. . . .

RECOMMENDED READING

The books outlined below are ones I've read and would recommend reading as part of your journey towards health. The science and research mentioned throughout *House-training the Diabetes Monster* are mainly a result of reading these books. The authors and people mentioned below have not endorsed this book, nor were they contacted for an endorsement. These books are merely my recommended reading list.

Why We Get fat - Gary Taubes

Good Calories Bad Calories - Gary Taubes

Fat Chance - Dr. Robert Lustig

Grain Brain - Dr. David Perlmutter

Brain Maker - Dr. David Perlmutter

The Hunger Fix – Dr. Pamela Peeke

Beat Sugar Addiction Now - Dr. Jacob Teitelbaum

From Fatigued to Fantastic - Dr. Jacob Teitelbaum

While Science Sleeps: A Sweetener Kills – Dr. Woodrow Monte

Gut and Psychology Syndrome - Dr. Natasha Campbell-McBride

The Obesity Epidemic: What Caused it? How Can We Stop It? - Zoe Harcombe

The Inflammation Cure - Dr. William Joel Meggs

How Your Mind Can Heal Your Body - Dana Hamilton, Ph.D.

The 4 Agreements - Don Miguel Ruiz

I Can See Clearly Now - Wayne Dyer

The Power of Story - Jim Loehr

Knockout - Suzanne Somers

PACE: Rediscover Your Native Fitness - Dr. Al Sears

GULP: Adventures on the Alimentary Canal - Mary Roach

The Great Cholesterol Con - Anthony Colpo

Integrative Nutrition - Joshua Rosenthal

Effortless Healing - Dr. Joseph Marcela

The Ultrasimple Diet - Dr. Mark Hyman

The Guide to Healthy Eating - Dr. David Brownstein

The Food-Mood Solution - Jack Challem

Junk Foods & Junk Moods - Lindsay Smith

Forget Fitting In - Jen Viano

Diabetes Epidemic & You - Dr. Joseph R. Kraft

Ending the War on Fat - Joy Bauer

Vitamin K2 and the Calcium Paradox: How a Little Known Vitamin Could Save Your Live - Dr. Kate Rheaume-Bleue

People and websites I follow online:

Dr. Joseph Mercola

Dr. Blaylock - The Blaylock Report

Dr. Andrew Weil

Dr. Mark Hyman

Authority Nutrition - Kris Gunners

The Diet Doctor